HEARTBEAT

A Complete Guide to Understanding and Preventing Heart Disease

HEARTBEAT

A Complete Guide to Understanding and Preventing Heart Disease

Emmanuel Horovitz, M.D.

Illustrations by Therese Trebaol

Health Trend Publishing, Los Angeles

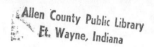
This book is available at special discounts with bulk purchases for educational or promotional use. For further information, please write to:

Health Trend Publishing
P.O. Box 17420
Encino, CA 91416-7420

Publisher's Cataloging in Publication Data

Horovitz, Emmanuel.

      Heartbeat: A Complete Guide to Understanding and Preventing Heart Disease.

      Includes Index.

1. Heart—Diseases—Popular works.
2. Coronary heart disease—Prevention.

        616.12   87-082715

ISBN 0-9619329-6-1 (softcover)

ISBN 0-9619329-5-3 (hardcover)

Health Trend Publishing
P.O Box 17420
Encino, CA 91416-7420

9 8 7 6 5 4 3 2 1

This book is designed to assist the reader to better understand heart disease, and is not intended to be a substitute for the medical advice and ongoing care of a personal physician. The reader should regularly consult his or her physician about matters relating to health, particularly regarding any symptoms that may require medical attention.

Contents

Acknowledgements

I would like to acknowledge and thank Dennis Cohen, Herm Perlmutter, and Ken Fisher, for their detailed review of the manuscript and for their useful suggestions. I also wish to thank Drs. Alex Greenberger and Robert Natelson for reading portions of the manuscript. Special thanks to my friend and colleague, Dr. Larry Whitfield, for his encouragement, and for introducing me to the fascinating world of the Macintosh.

My sincere appreciation to Therese Trebaol for providing the artwork, and for her dedication to this project. My appreciation to Marshal Licht, Chuck and Heidi Wiedeman, and Graphics Plus, for their help in the various aspects of the production of this book.

My thanks are due to the following people who have helped me in so many different ways: Robert Baral, Susan Shell, Dr. Tony Greenberg, Dan Poynter, Jan Nathan, Terry Sherf, and Robert Erdmann.

Special thanks are expressed to Linda Rook, my office manager, for her indispensable help and for her understanding.

And last, but not least, my deep and sincere appreciation to Rachel Grant for her help in initiating this project, and for her continuous support and encouragement during the various stages of the project.

Preface

Very often, people who suffer a heart attack or are diagnosed as having heart disease are both stunned and frightened. Naturally, they are concerned about how their condition will affect them and their loved ones. They may wonder: Will I come out of this all right? Will I be able to keep my job? Will it affect my marriage and my sex life? Will I be able to play tennis again? Must I give up all those delicious foods that contain butter and cream? Will I need bypass surgery?

Today, more than ever, people are deeply concerned with matters of personal health, and are determined to take charge of their own well-being. But first, they need answers to their questions — they need information! Unfortunately, relevant medical information is often buried in lengthy, complicated medical textbooks and is expressed in complex medical jargon. The doctor, of course, could spend hours answering all these important questions, but where is he going to get the time?

As a practicing cardiologist, I realized, a few years back, that there was a need for a well-written book about heart disease, a book that would answer in detail these and other relevant questions patients have. I therefore decided to write a comprehensive, yet readable guidebook about heart disease, addressed to patients and their families as well as to lay readers and educators. The task was not easy because of the vast amount of material that needed to be covered, and the difficulty of "translating" medical jargon into layman's terms. After several years of work, I believe I have met the challenge and written a book that accomplishes these goals.

The main purpose of *Heartbeat* is to describe the essential features of various types of heart disease in readable language, not so that patients will become medical experts, but rather to help patients understand the nature of their disease, its treatment, and its prevention. This type of information should help them ask relevant questions, and therefore help break some of the communication barriers that often exist between patients and their doctors. Also, by learning the various symptoms of heart disease, perhaps people will seek medical help at an earlier stage, before the advent of a major cardiac event, such as a heart attack or bypass surgery.

Although heart disease still remains the major cause of disability and death in this country, the death rate from heart disease has been steadily declining. Evidence indicates that this is due, at least in part, to preventive measures, such as giving up smoking, eating a proper diet, and exercising regularly. An important goal of this book, therefore, is to discuss the various risk factors for heart disease, and provide simple and practical guidelines for prevention. By promoting prudent health habits and sensible lifestyles we could, to some extent, prevent unnecessary illness, needless loss of vitality, and premature death.

In order to make the book more readable, I have tried to be as clear and straightforward as possible. Technical data usually expressed in complex medical jargon have been translated into layman's terms. In addition, numerous graphs and illustrations accompany the text.

To make this book easier to understand, I have chosen to discuss only facts and data relevant to the understanding of the disease process and its management. For this reason, I have not discussed certain procedures used only in a very small number of patients (such as heart transplants, artificial hearts); procedures that are still at an experimental stage (such as coronary laser angioplasty); and treatments that have not shown to have any proven benefits (such as chelation therapy).

As a physician, I have always enjoyed the challenge of answering patients' questions as completely and as clearly as possible. I hope *Heartbeat* will provide answers to the many questions patients have about heart disease, and will motivate people of all ages to achieve a better, healthier lifestyle.

Part One

PREVENTING
HEART DISEASE

1 Heart Disease: Today's Great Challenge

Despite numerous advances and a decade of declining death rates, heart disease remains the leading cause of disability and death in the United States and other industrialized nations. This year alone, as many as 1,500,000 Americans will suffer a heart attack, and over a third of them will die from it. Heart disease is not only a disease of the elderly; it often afflicts men and women in the prime of life, during their most productive years.

Coronary heart disease, the most common form of heart disease, is due to the accumulation of fatty deposits in the walls of the coronary arteries (the arteries feeding the heart muscle). The underlying condition, called atherosclerosis, is a degenerative process that involves arteries in the heart, brain, and other parts of the body. The lining of the arteries becomes thickened and roughened by deposits of fat, cholesterol, cellular debris, and calcium. The process begins early in life, as early as childhood, and then progresses slowly over the years. As these deposits (called plaques) continue to build up, the inside of the arteries become narrowed, thus slowing down the flow of blood.

The presence of mild or even moderate narrowing of the coronary arteries is generally not associated with any symptoms. Over the years, however, when one or more of the coronary arteries become severely narrowed by an enlarging plaque, symptoms eventually occur. The clinical manifestations of coronary heart disease are multiple and varied. Some patients, for example, may suffer from recurrent chest pain (angina) due to inadequate delivery of blood to the heart muscle. Others may suffer permanent damage to an area of the heart muscle (heart attack or myocardial infarction) resulting from the total blockage of a coronary artery. Finally, sudden death may be the initial and only manifestation of coronary heart disease, and it often occurs without any prior warning.

Another common form of cardiovascular (pertaining to the heart and blood vessels) disease is high blood pressure, or hypertension, a condition characterized by an excessive amount of pressure within the arteries. High blood pressure is the most common chronic medical problem in this country today, affecting over 20 percent of the adult population. A chronic elevation of the blood pressure leads to an acceleration of the atherosclerotic process, that is, the deposit of fatty plaques in the walls of the arteries. This process is especially common in the major arterial branches conducting blood to the heart and brain. Indeed, hypertensive patients have a significant increase in the risk of developing heart attacks and strokes.

Less common forms of heart disease include disorders of the heart valves, diseases of the heart muscle, and congenital heart defects. In each group, the clinical manifestations are extremely variable, ranging from minor symptoms to severe disability and threat to life. Two relatively common conditions, congestive heart failure and cardiac arrhythmias (disturbances of the heart rhythm), can result from a wide variety of cardiovascular diseases. The term "heart failure" does not mean imminent death from heart disease; it simply implies that the pumping function of the heart is impaired. Cardiac arrhythmias result from disturbances in the cardiac electrical system, and they sometimes occur in persons with an otherwise perfectly normal heart.

Some Good News. . .

Until this century, infectious diseases (such as tuberculosis, diphtheria, and smallpox) were the major killers. Since around 1930, however, diseases of the heart and blood vessels have replaced infectious diseases as the leading cause of death in the United States. Yet, a look at the age-adjusted death rates reveals a 30 percent decline in cardiovascular mortality beginning in the 1950s (see figure 1). Nearly two thirds of this decline has occurred since around 1970. Although the exact reasons for the decline in death rates are not well defined, it appears to be related to two major factors: a) the improvement in medical care, and b) the changes in lifestyle of the American people.

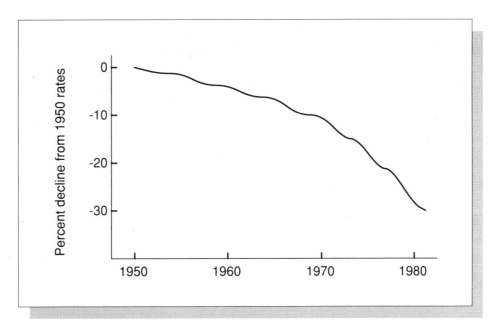

Figure 1. Percent decline in age-adjusted death rate for cardiovascular diseases, United States, 1950 to 1980.

Over the past twenty years, there has been a substantial improvement in the quality of medical care given to patients with heart disease. Emergency medical services are better equipped to treat coronary patients, and training in cardiopulmonary resuscitation is more widespread. The use of specialized coronary care units has reduced the mortality from life-threatening cardiac arrhythmias during the first few hours after a heart attack. The development and use of sophisticated techniques and procedures has enhanced our capacity to detect and diagnose various types of heart disease, and allowed us to do this at an earlier stage of the disease. The use of new cardiovascular drugs has improved our ability to control certain conditions such as angina, congestive heart failure, high blood pressure, and cardiac arrhythmias. Finally, the development of coronary bypass surgery and coronary balloon angioplasty has improved the life expectancy of many patients with severe coronary heart disease.

Studies have shown that certain traits or habits, termed "risk factors," are associated with an increased likelihood of developing coronary heart disease. Several of these risk factors are classified as controllable, meaning they can be changed or treated. Among these controllable risk factors are cigarette smoking, high blood cholesterol, obesity, and high blood pressure. It is likely that changes in the lifestyle of the American people over the past two decades have contributed to the decline in the death rate from heart disease. Today, Americans are more aware of maintaining their health: they smoke less, exercise more, consume less fat, and monitor their weight and blood pressure better than they did twenty years ago.

At this time, no one can say for sure what part, either improved medical care or changes in lifestyle, have played in the declining mortality from heart disease. Until a cause and effect relationship can be clearly demonstrated, we may not be able to decide the extent to which treatment or prevention is responsible for the decline. Fortunately though, more advances are being made in both areas than ever before.

. . . and Some Bad News

Despite the recent decline in mortality rates, cardiovascular diseases still account for nearly half of all deaths in this country (see figure 2). Most of the technology available today is directed toward managing the problem of heart disease after it has occurred. This approach, although effective in many cases, does not deal with the underlying cause of coronary heart disease, that is, the build-up of fatty plaques within the coronary arteries. Antianginal drugs, for example, can relieve symptoms of angina, but they do not slow down the progression of atherosclerosis. Coronary bypass surgery and coronary balloon angioplasty are effective in relieving angina and prolonging the life of many patients. These procedures, however, are only palliative measures that "buy time," while coronary heart disease is a chronic and progressive condition.

The results of technological progress have undeniably brought benefits to millions of patients, but the benefits of progress have been mixed with some negative aspects. The very existence of sophisticated medical technology may lead to its excessive use, and this can in turn lead to sky-

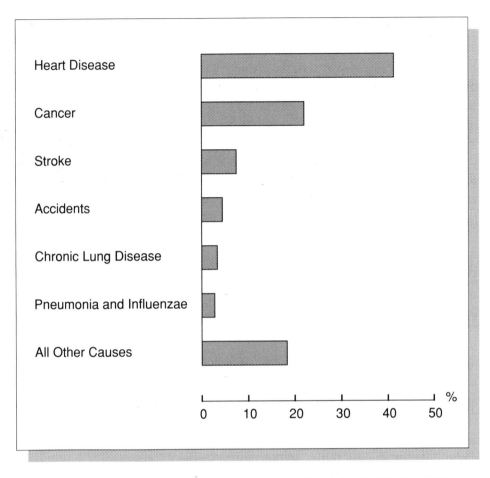

Figure 2. Deaths by cause, as percentage of total deaths (U.S., 1983).

rocketing costs. Also, in our society, a high level of prestige is attached to fast, dramatic actions based on technological solutions, as opposed to slow, gradual progress based on education. Patients often reinforce this unbalanced emphasis; they expect a "cure" for every ache and stress. In such a society, it is not surprising that doctors prefer to quickly diagnose and cure, and are less enthusiastic about patient problems that may require gradual education and counseling.

The Challenge

In view of the recent decline in the death rate from cardiovascular diseases, it is reasonable to believe that we can control, to some extent, the process of atherosclerosis and its major complications (heart attacks and strokes). The success of such an endeavor will depend on the progress made on several fronts, especially ongoing medical research, improved medical and surgical care, public education, and changes in personal lifestyle.

As we become involved with a more and more sophisticated technology, it is important to remember that such developments are based on knowledge and understanding. We must continue improving our knowledge by devoting more time to, and providing more funds for, medical research.

In the last decade, there has been tremendous growth in our understanding of the basic process of atherosclerosis and its major cardiovascular consequences. Much more research is needed, however, before we can define the real impact of various sophisticated diagnostic and therapeutic procedures (such as computerized imaging techniques, coronary bypass surgery, and coronary balloon angioplasty) on the progression of the disease. Although the evidence strongly suggests that changes in lifestyle have a beneficial effect, more research is required before we can define the relative contribution of each factor, and prove the existence of a cause and effect relationship.

Over the past two decades, there have been tremendous technological advances in medicine, especially in the field of cardiology. We must realize, however, that the advances in medical technology have been somewhat uneven, and that the positive benefits of progress are mixed with some negative results. In addressing these issues, we should not ignore or underestimate the real benefits of this progress. Improved technology has undoubtedly brought benefits to millions of cardiac patients by prolonging and saving many lives. What is needed, however, is a critical assessment of the various technological advances, and the application of constructive adjustments. When dealing with the individual patient, physicians must use sound clinical judgement based on common sense and understanding, rather than be tempted by the abundant availability of sophisticated diagnostic and therapeutic procedures.

It is clear that despite all the improvements in medical and surgical care, we cannot rely entirely on repair and palliation. It is therefore reasonable to suggest an active approach to lifestyle changes and risk factor modification as a way of preventing coronary heart disease. By making changes in their own lifestyle (giving up smoking, eating a proper diet, and exercising regularly), individuals can modify or even eliminate these risk factors, and therefore be in a position to prevent, or at least delay, the progression of coronary heart disease. Voluntary health organizations, such as the American Heart Association, have had a major role in promoting public education and community service programs. It may well be that the decline in mortality from heart disease is at least in part the result of these improved health habits of the general public.

An important ingredient in patient education is a better doctor-patient relationship, based on effective communication and trust. The doctor must make an effort to explain the nature of the condition in a language that the patient can understand, avoiding complex medical jargon, and answering questions willingly and clearly. Printed educational materials given to patients can provide a convenient reference for patients and families, stimulate relevant questions, and reduce anxiety.

Patients also have responsibilities. In order to claim a share in the decision making, they must educate themselves by reading educational materials and by asking appropriate questions. They must also take the important preventive measures that only they can take, such as giving up smoking, acquiring healthier eating habits, and exercising regularly. People generally feel better when they understand what the problem is, and when they realize they can promote their own health by making real changes in their habits and lifestyle.

2 Risk Factors for Heart Disease

Risk factors are those conditions and habits associated with an increased risk or likelihood of an individual developing coronary heart disease (the most prevalent form of heart disease). A person with one or more risk factors is more likely to experience angina or suffer a heart attack, and he will do so at a relatively younger age. When two or more major risk factors are present simultaneously, the risk is multiplied.

It should be emphasized, however, that not everyone having one or more risk factors will actually develop heart disease. Conversely, heart disease will sometimes develop in persons with no risk factors at all. Also, no definite scientific data exist to prove that elimination or correction of risk factors can reverse the atherosclerotic process and cause actual regression of the already existing plaques.

The knowledge of risk factors is helpful in assessing the risk of the individual for developing coronary heart disease, provided that he does not already have evidence of the disease. In other words, if a person does already have manifestations of coronary heart disease (such as recurrent symptoms of angina, history of a heart attack), the knowledge of risk factors is of little value in assessing the risk. A 40-year-old athlete suffering from typical chest pains on exertion, for example, should not ignore his symptoms just because he is an "unlikely candidate." This person could conceivably have significant coronary heart disease even though he does not smoke, has a normal blood pressure, and eats a proper diet!

Certain risk factors are classified as uncontrollable, meaning they cannot be changed or modified. These include the person's age, sex, and heredity. Among the controllable (or treatable) risk factors, three are

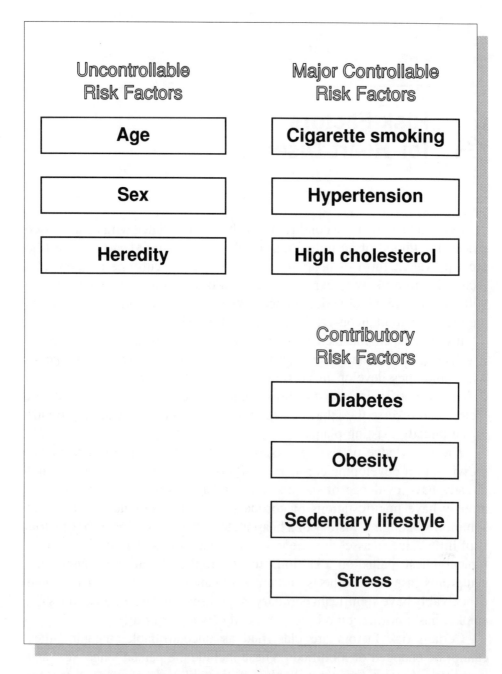

Figure 3. Risk factors for coronary heart disease.

thought to be most important in the development of atherosclerosis: cigarette smoking, high blood pressure, and elevated blood cholesterol level. Additional contributing risk factors are: diabetes, obesity, lack of physical activity, and personality type.

Uncontrollable Risk Factors

Age

Although heart disease is not caused by aging per se, it is more common among older people. In general, the longer a person lives, the greater his chances of developing the disease. It has been demonstrated that atherosclerosis begins at an early age, then progresses slowly over the years, often without any manifestations. It then becomes a major cause of morbidity and mortality for persons in their fifties and sixties.

Sex

Statistics have shown that men have a higher incidence of coronary heart disease than women in the same age range. The fact that women are less likely to develop the disease is probably due to the presence of natural female sex hormones, which appear to protect against the build-up of plaques within the arteries. Following menopause, women "catch up" with men, and by the age of sixty they develop the disease at a similar rate. It is interesting to note that in recent years, women have become afflicted earlier in life and in greater numbers than in the past. A possible explanation is that women now smoke more, have entered the competitive job market in greater numbers, and are subjected to the same stresses as their male counterparts.

Heredity

It has been shown that persons whose parents, uncles, or siblings were victims of angina or heart attack at a relatively young age (in their forties and fifties) are at greater risk of developing the disease themselves. In addition to the inherited genetic influence, the home environment may play a role. Studies have shown, for example, that when both parents smoke, their children are more likely to smoke too, later in life. Although family history cannot be changed, steps can be taken to minimize the chances of coronary heart disease by identifying and then changing the risk factors at an early age.

Major Controllable Risk Factors

Cigarette Smoking

There is substantial evidence linking cigarette smoking to the risk of atherosclerosis and coronary heart disease. A variety of mechanisms have been suggested to explain the adverse effects of cigarette smoking on the heart and blood vessels. (For more information on smoking, see Chapter 3). Persons who smoke a pack of cigarettes a day, for example, have more than twice the risk of having a heart attack than nonsmokers. In general, the risk is directly proportional to the number of cigarettes smoked.

Persons who give up smoking have a lesser risk of coronary heart disease than those who continue to smoke. In fact, once the habit is given up, the risk gradually declines toward the same level as that of people who have never smoked. Within two years after quitting, for example, the risk of a heart attack in formers smokers is about half that of smokers. After ten years the risk is lowered to practically the same level as for those who have never smoked.

High Blood Pressure

High blood pressure, also termed hypertension, is an excessive amount of pressure within the arteries. A chronic elevation of the blood pressure leads to an acceleration of the atherosclerotic process, that is, the deposit of fatty plaques in the walls of the arteries. This process is especially common in the major arterial branches conducting blood to vital organs, such as the heart, brain, and kidneys. High blood pressure also increases the resistance to blood flow in the arteries, thus causing an increased workload on the heart. (For more information on high blood pressure, see Chapter 15).

An elevated blood pressure is associated with an increased risk of developing coronary heart disease as well as other cardiovascular complications, such as congestive heart failure and strokes. There is no specific point at which the risk suddenly changes from low to high values. In other words, the higher the blood pressure, the higher the risk of developing cardiovascular diseases.

The reduction of blood pressure through treatment has been shown to protect against cardiovascular complications. In fact, several studies have shown that treatment of moderate or severe hypertension significantly reduces the incidence of heart attacks, congestive heart failure, and strokes. Any effective treatment program for high blood pressure must include certain changes in diet and lifestyle (such as restriction of salt, weight loss, and regular exercise) whether or not drug therapy is later required.

High Blood Cholesterol Level

Cholesterol is a fatty yellow material that is normally present in the blood. It is manufactured by the liver as part of the normal process of digestion. Cholesterol is found in many of the foods we eat, such as eggs, meat, chicken, fish, and dairy products. Although our body needs a certain amount of cholesterol, an excessive amount can be harmful, because the extra cholesterol can deposit and build up in the walls of the arteries, and can lead to the acceleration of the atherosclerotic process. Cholesterol and the other fats, the triglycerides, do not circulate freely in the blood, but are transported in the form of lipoprotein complexes — large molecules combining lipids (fats) and proteins.

Depending on their relative composition in cholesterol, triglycerides, and protein, the lipoprotein complexes can be classified into several types. They are often classified by their size or density as determined by chemical means. Most of the cholesterol in the blood is carried in a specific type of lipoproteins, called Low Density Lipoproteins (or LDL). The LDL complexes are responsible for transporting the cholesterol to the body cells. An elevated level of LDL will increase fatty build-up in the arteries, and will therefore contribute to premature development of atherosclerosis. Multiple studies have shown a direct correlation between the level of LDL cholesterol and the risk of coronary heart disease. No correlation has been found, however, between the blood level of triglycerides and the incidence of coronary heart disease.

The blood level of cholesterol varies among individuals, and depends on several factors, including heredity, sex, and age. In the United States, the

Age	"High Risk" Level	Desirable Level
20 - 29	Greater than 220	Lower than 160
30 - 39	Greater than 240	Lower than 180
40 and over	Greater than 260	Lower than 200

Figure 4. Blood cholesterol values (mg/dl) considered to be "high risk" for coronary heart disease, and the desirable levels.

average cholesterol level is about 220 milligrams per deciliter (mg/dl), a figure that is probably too high for optimal health (see figure 4). There is no "safe" level of cholesterol; as blood cholesterol decreases, so does the risk of developing atherosclerosis. In other words, the lower the cholesterol level, the better it is. One study showed that the relative incidence of coronary heart disease in middle-aged persons with cholesterol levels greater than 260 mg/dl was three to five times that of individuals with cholesterol levels of less than 220 mg/dl.

There appears to be a correlation between the type of diet a person eats and his level of cholesterol. Diets high in cholesterol (such as egg yolks, red meat, organ meats) or saturated fats (meat, butter, dairy products) tend to raise the blood level of cholesterol, whereas diets high in unsaturated fats (vegetable oils, margarine) tend to keep it low. In countries with a high standard of living, where diets rich in animal fats prevail, the levels of blood cholesterol are generally higher and the risk of heart disease is increased as compared to poorer countries where vegetarian-type diets predominate.

Cholesterol is also present in other types of lipoproteins, such as the High Density Lipoproteins (or HDL). The function of the HDL complexes is to remove cholesterol from the body cells and deliver it to the liver and other sites where it can be metabolized and eliminated. By their action, HDLs appear to actually protect the arteries against atherosclerosis.

Research has shown an inverse relationship between the concentration of HDL cholesterol (the so-called "good cholesterol") and the risk of coronary heart disease. In other words, individuals with higher levels of HDL tend to have a lower risk of coronary heart disease.

The higher the ratio of HDL to LDL cholesterol, the better. Factors that influence the HDL to LDL ratio include heredity, sex, exercise, diet, and cigarette smoking. Regular exercise activity, for example, tends to increase the HDL and lower the LDL cholesterol (that's good). Cigarette smoking, on the other hand, tends to lower the HDL and increase the LDL cholesterol (that's bad).

Contributory Risk Factors

Diabetes

Diabetes mellitus (or "sugar diabetes") is a condition in which the blood sugar level is abnormally elevated. Diabetes may be caused either by insufficient insulin or by the body's inability to use effectively the insulin it produces. Insulin is a hormone produced by the pancreas and used by the body to metabolize sugar and other carbohydrates. When an insufficient amount of insulin is produced, sugar accumulates in the blood.

Multiple studies have clearly shown that patients suffering from diabetes have a much higher risk of developing atherosclerosis than do nondiabetics. Diabetic patients have an increased frequency of heart attacks, strokes, and peripheral vascular disease (poor circulation to the legs). Those who develop diabetes at an early age are at greater risk than those in whom the disease occurs in later years.

The mechanisms associating diabetes and increased risk of coronary heart disease are not well understood yet. Higher levels of blood sugar increase the cholesterol level to a degree that may cause premature atherosclerosis. Also, many diabetic patients suffer from obesity and high blood pressure, two additional risk factors. Although diabetes can be brought under control with proper diet, weight reduction, and drugs (insulin injections, pills), it is not certain whether "tight" control of the blood sugar levels will ultimately result in a significantly lower risk of coronary heart disease in the individual diabetic patient.

Obesity

Obesity results from excess of fatty tissue in the body. The cutoff point between "normal" and "obese" can only be approximated, but it is generally defined as a 20 percent excess over ideal body weight. Tables of "ideal" or "desirable" body weight are based on estimates of what is consistent with a normal life expectancy. Such tables, often issued by life insurance companies, are more useful when adjusted for differences in body build. When using the above criteria of 20 percent excess weight, as many as 30 percent of the American people are considered obese!

Several studies have shown that the risk of developing coronary heart disease is higher in obese persons. Excess weight may not directly affect the heart itself, but it does certainly intensify several other risk factors. Indeed, obesity increases a person's chance of developing high blood pressure, elevated blood cholesterol, and diabetes. Therefore, achieving and maintaining a desirable body weight will generally have a beneficial effect on blood pressure, blood cholesterol, and blood sugar levels.

Lack of Physical Activity

In our society, the extended use of mechanical energy to replace human physical energy has led to increased physical inactivity and a sedentary lifestyle. There is little question that these changes in mobility and effort have had an undesirable effect on total body fitness and on the tendency toward obesity.

The role of exercise in the prevention of heart disease has become a subject of increasing interest to both the general public and medical researchers. Several studies have shown a statistical link between a sedentary lifestyle and increased incidence of coronary heart disease. Other investigations have shown, although not conclusively, that an exercise training program may decrease the chances of sustaining a heart attack. Such studies are difficult to perform on a large scale because of the influence of multiple variables and other risk factors. For instance, persons who do not exercise regularly are often overweight, have an elevated blood pressure, and are more likely to smoke cigarettes.

Several theories exist regarding the role of exercise in providing "protection" against heart disease. First of all, regular exercise results in "conditioning" of the heart and the circulatory system, meaning it improves the efficiency of oxygen utilization by the heart, lungs, and body muscles. Another theory suggests that exercise causes the development of small new blood vessels within the heart muscle, termed collateral circulation, thus providing better blood flow to the heart muscle. If this is true, such blood vessels would serve as emergency short-circuits and compensate for the loss in blood supply in case of a blockage of a large coronary artery (myocardial infarction or heart attack).

Regular exercise can also help reduce several other risk factors, such as high blood pressure, high blood cholesterol level, and obesity. Patients who exercise, for example, tend to have a lower blood pressure and a slower heart rate. With exercise training, there is often a reduction in the level of triglycerides and cholesterol in the blood, as well as an elevation of the High Density Lipoprotein (HDL, the "good cholesterol"). Along with a proper diet, exercise is helpful in burning excess calories and reducing body weight. Finally, many smokers give up their habit after they start exercising, particularly when they choose an exercise they enjoy.

Stress and Personality Type

In general terms, stress occurs when there exists an imbalance between excessive environmental demands and the person's ability to cope with them. If recurrent or prolonged, stress may harm the person's health and well-being. Not all stress, however, is necessarily bad or detrimental. All of us need a certain amount of stress to add variety and spice to life, to prod us to achieve goals. Some people even thrive on stress; they find working under pressure or against deadlines highly stimulating.

The relationship between stress and coronary heart disease does not appear to be a direct cause and effect, but rather the result of a complex process affecting the body's systems. It has been suggested that the effects of stress on the cardiovascular system operate through the release of certain hormones (such as adrenaline) by the adrenal glands. The release of these substances in turn induces a series of events, which include acceleration of the heart rate, rise of the blood pressure, and pouring of fatty substances into the bloodstream, all factors in the development of atherosclerosis and coronary heart disease.

In recent years, a good deal has been written about the possible role of personality type in causing heart disease. Much of this stems from the research of two San Francisco physicians, Drs. Friedman and Rosenman. After interviewing a large number of heart attack patients, they began to see a common behavior pattern, which they termed "Type A behavior," in many of these patients. They concluded that a person with a hard-driven and time-conscious personality (Type A) is at a higher risk of developing a heart attack than a person who is calm and easy-going (Type B).

Typically, a Type A person is competitive, shows a sense of urgency about time, and has an unrelenting determination to forge ahead quickly both socially and economically. In other words, this is a person who wants to do too many things in too little time. The Type A person is often a "workaholic" who takes little, if any, time to relax for fear of falling behind. He may be quick-tempered, compulsive, suspicious, and even hostile. The excessive drive to meet career and personal goals generally produces a great deal of emotional stress, which can result in elevation of the blood pressure. In contrast, the Type B person is more relaxed, less competitive, and not so driven by time and the need to succeed.

The possible association between personality type and the risk of coronary heart disease is still the subject of continuing controversy. A few studies have found that Type A men had twice the risk of developing coronary heart disease as did Type B men. Other large-scale studies, however, have not confirmed these findings.

Regardless of the roots of Type A behavior, an important question is whether or not attempts should be made to modify it! In our success-oriented, competitive society, the Type A person is rewarded by achieving many of the goals that we hold in such high esteem: money, status, and power, among others. Furthermore, most Type A persons seem to enjoy their hectic, fast-paced lives and have no desire to change. They prefer to think of themselves as competent and competitive rather than "compulsive" and "hostile;" as conscientious and productive rather than "time-slaves" and "workaholics."

Risk Factor Modification

The fact that some risk factors can be changed should be regarded as good news. By making changes in their own lifestyle — giving up smoking, eating a proper diet, and exercising regularly — individuals can modify or even eliminate these risk factors, and therefore be in a position to prevent, or at least delay, the progression of coronary heart disease.

Several risk factors (such as high blood pressure, high cholesterol level, and diabetes) do not cause any symptoms during their early stages (they are termed "silent"). For this reason, adults are urged to have regular screenings for these conditions. The initial checkup should begin at age 20 and be repeated at least every five years. In addition, a blood pressure reading should be obtained every year or two, because blood pressure can creep up unexpectedly. Older people may need a medical checkup at more frequent intervals. Checkups are particularly important if there is a family history of heart disease, high blood pressure, high cholesterol level, or diabetes. It is the responsibility of individuals to make an appointment with their physician and to insist on risk factor screening.

Remember!

Atherosclerosis is a slow progressive disease that begins early in life, as early as childhood. All too often, patients wait until the occurrence of a major cardiac event (such as heart attack or coronary bypass surgery) before making the necessary adjustments. It would make better sense to begin the changes in lifestyle early enough, before the disease has reached an advanced stage. In fact, there is no better time to start a new healthy lifestyle than today!

It may be helpful to regard these preventive measures as a personal investment that, if wisely attended to, can only have a positive return. There is no guarantee that modification of risk factors in the individual person will indeed prevent the development of heart disease. These measures, however, will result in better general health and improved physical fitness, and will contribute to an increased sense of well-being.

③ Giving Up the Smoking Habit

"Warning: The Surgeon General Has Determined That Cigarette Smoking is Dangerous to Your Health." A warning label similar to this one now appears on every pack of cigarettes. Since the Surgeon General's landmark report in 1964, the percentage of smokers in the population has been declining. While this is encouraging, there are about 50 million Americans who still smoke cigarettes today, comprising approximately 35 percent of adult males and 30 percent of adult females.

The Hazards of Smoking

Cigarette smoking is one of the three major risk factors for the development of coronary heart disease. Persons who smoke one pack of cigarettes a day have more than twice the risk of suffering a heart attack than do non-smokers. Cigarette smoking may interact negatively with other risk factors as well. When combined with both high blood pressure and high cholesterol levels, for example, the risk of developing coronary heart disease becomes ten times that of a "low-risk" individual! Smokers can expect a shorter life span than nonsmokers. As an example, the life expectancy of a 25-year-old who smokes two packs a day is about 8 years shorter than that of a nonsmoker.

Cigarette smoking is also the leading cause of chronic lung disease, chronic bronchitis, and emphysema. Smoking is the number one cause of lung cancer, and a major cause of mouth and throat cancer. In smokers there is a progressive decline of respiratory function and a reduction of exercise tolerance, even before any manifestations of disease appear.

SURGEON GENERAL'S WARNING: Smoking Causes
Heart Disease, Lung Cancer, and Emphysema

Cigarette smoking is associated with a certain degree of addiction to *nicotine*, a powerful drug found in tobacco. As smoke is inhaled, nicotine passes through the membrane of the lung tissue and rapidly enters the bloodstream. Then, within ten seconds, the inhaled nicotine reaches the brain, where it induces the release of adrenaline-like substances, called catecholamines. The effect of these substances is to accelerate the heart rate and raise the blood pressure. These changes in the body's metabolism are the "lift" that smokers crave.

Addicted smokers must keep a continuous amount of nicotine circulating in the blood and going to the brain. If that amount falls below a certain level or if they stop smoking, they may experience unpleasant withdrawal symptoms. Symptoms of withdrawal may include the following: headache, nausea, fatigue, drowsiness, insomnia, inability to concentrate, irritability, anxiety, depression, and craving for cigarettes. Smokers who try to quit should be prepared to accept withdrawal symptoms as a natural consequence of stopping. Withdrawal is a temporary condition that, though unpleasant with some people, is not harmful.

In addition to nicotine, cigarette smoke contains harmful gases. There exist many such gases, but the most dangerous one is *carbon monoxide*, a colorless and odorless gas. Carbon monoxide has a stronger attraction (by 200 times!) for red blood cells than does oxygen. Since red blood cells are meant to carry oxygen throughout the body, this means that carbon monoxide is replacing oxygen, therefore interfering with the distribution of oxygen to the body cells.

Carbon monoxide seems to be nicotine's accomplice in many assaults on the smoker's body. Studies have shown that carbon monoxide makes it easier for fatty substances to pass through the walls of arteries. This may be one of the mechanisms leading to acceleration of atherosclerosis, that is, the build-up of fatty plaques within the arteries. The adrenaline released by jolts of inhaled nicotine aids this process by affecting fat cells all over the body, causing them to pour fatty acids into the bloodstream. Every time a person smokes, the blood level of these fatty acids increases.

Elevated levels of fatty acids may also have a harmful effect on the blood clotting process. Some studies have shown that the platelets (tiny corpuscles that participate in the clotting mechanism) become more adhesive (sticky) in smokers. This may explain why smokers get more heart attacks than nonsmokers — their blood more readily forms clots, which may block a coronary artery, thereby causing a heart attack.

In addition to nicotine and harmful gases, cigarette smoke also contains *tars*, that is, solid chemical particles which, when inhaled, condense as sticky substances in the lungs. These tars interfere with the normal function of the lungs and may result in lung disease. Indeed, smoking is the leading cause of emphysema, an irreversible condition which reduces the lung's elasticity and destroys the air sacs, thereby reducing the amount of lung surface available for the exchange of oxygen. A number of chemicals present in tar are known to produce cancer. Cancers begin when tars produce abnormal cells in the mouth, throat, and lungs; these irregular cells then develop into tumors.

The damage done by cigarettes is "dose related," meaning that each cigarette does some harm. Each additional inhalation then increases the damage. There is no such thing as a safe level of smoking, nor such a thing as a safe cigarette. Research has shown that cutting down on the number of cigarettes smoked, as well as smoking those which have efficient filters and less tar and nicotine, may reduce the risk of serious illness. However, cutting down is not the best way to go for people who really want to avoid the dangers of smoking. The only certain way to do this (and for the great majority of smokers, the easiest way) is to quit smoking altogether.

There is no doubt that cigarette smoking is a health hazard of the first order. The good news, however, is that many of the adverse effects of smoking can be reversed. Ex-smokers have a lower risk of developing

SURGEON GENERAL'S WARNING: Quitting Smoking Now Greatly Reduces Serious Risks to Your Health coronary heart disease than those who continue to smoke. Once the habit is given up, the risk gradually declines over the years. Studies have shown that within two years after quitting, the risk of a heart attack in former smokers is about half the risk in smokers. After ten years, the risk is practically the same as for nonsmokers!

Smokers themselves are not the only ones affected by tobacco smoke. Although the evidence so far is not as conclusive as it is for smokers, nonsmokers exposed to tobacco (for example, nonsmokers married to smokers) may also be at risk. Several studies suggest a positive relationship between so-called "passive (or involuntary) smoking" and the incidence of lung cancer.

Approaches to Quitting Smoking

Those who want to quit smoking can take heart in the fact that more than 30 million people have done so successfully since the Surgeon's General Report on Smoking in 1964. Although smoking cessation programs of one kind or another are helpful for some, most people who stop do so on their own. Motivation appears to be the key element in many of the success stories. No one method of quitting works for everyone: some stop "cold turkey," while others cut down gradually. Many smokers are helped by joining low-cost smoking cessation clinics.

With a *self-help program*, smokers are provided with brochures, books, audio tapes, and kits that will lead them through a program of smoking cessation on their own. A variety of voluntary organizations (such as the American Lung Association, the American Heart Association, and the American Cancer Society) offer helpful literature and various materials for smokers who try to give up the habit.

A number of organizations, public and private, hold low-cost *smoking cessation clinics* that treat smoking in a group format. Programs consist of a series of meetings for about one to two hours each. Usually included are lectures, inspirational messages, films, and group interaction. Other methods for smoking cessation include individual and group counseling, hypnosis, and behavior modification.

Probably the most effective strategy is to choose a specific date in the future, and when that date arrives, quit "*cold turkey.*" The first few days are the most difficult, when the various withdrawal symptoms (previously described) may occur. After that, the physiological and psychological needs gradually begin to lessen.

Another strategy, somewhat less effective, is the *step-by-step method*. Some may use progressively stronger filters or switch to cigarette brands of lower tar and nicotine content. Others may adopt such measures as delaying lighting up, inhaling smoke fewer times, laying down the cigarette for certain lengths of time between puffs, and extinguishing the cigarette after smoking it for only a short time.

Another method is based on the use of *nicotine substitutes*. The alternate substance is extracted from the leaves of tobacco plants, and then used in the form of chewing gum or tablet. This option appears to counter the urge to smoke and thus eases the smoker through the period of withdrawal. Nicotine substitutes are sold in drugstores under a variety of brand names (such as Nicorette®).

The rewards of giving up smoking are considerable. Often, there is an increased feeling of well-being. There may be a gradual improvement in stamina, and a slow disappearance of the hacking "cigarette cough." The socially undesirable features of cigarette smoking (such as bad breath, stained teeth, stained fingers, and cigarette odor in clothes) fade away rapidly. Most importantly, the potential risk of developing coronary heart disease and lung disease steadily declines over a period of several years.

Smoking Habits and Quitting

Most smokers begin to smoke in their teenage years. Peer pressure may be necessary for those first cigarettes, since the sensations are mostly unpleasant in the beginning. Smoking becomes a learned behavior. For most people, the first step in quitting is an awareness and identification of their smoking habits and a conscious effort to replace old habits with new ones.

Some smokers smoke for the *stimulant* effect; it gives them a "lift" or appears to get them going. They are likely to begin the day with a cigarette. They may want to smoke more when they feel tired, and get a "kick" out of smoking. Instead of a cigarette, these smokers can take a brisk walk, do a few stretches at their desk, or just open the window and breathe fresh air.

Smoking is sometimes used to occupy the hands, or for the pleasure of *handling* the paraphernalia of cigarettes. Smokers may have certain rituals about smoking: the kind of pack they prefer, the way they take out the cigarette, and the way they light it up with matches or a lighter. They probably enjoy watching the smoke, perhaps blowing smoke rings, or exhaling through the nose. Instead of a cigarette, smokers can substitute other objects to keep their hands busy, such as a pen or a pencil, a coin, "worry beads," or some other harmless object.

Some people use smoking in order to *relax*, as a reward for getting a job done, and to enhance the pleasures of eating, driving a car, or conversation. Chances are they most enjoy smoking after a meal, a cocktail, or coffee. These smokers often find that an honest consideration of the harmful effects of their habit is enough to help them quit. They may substitute social activities, exercise, eating (in moderation), and find they do not seriously miss their cigarettes.

Others smoke to *ease times of stress*, when they are anxious, angry, or upset. For them a cigarette is like a tranquilizer. Smokers who use smoking as this kind of coping mechanism will have to face the fact that cigarettes do not resolve the conditions that produce stress. Finding a substitute activity can help many through their difficult moments. Again, social activities, exercise, or eating may serve as useful substitutes for cigarettes even in times of "stress."

Some smokers reach for a cigarette merely out of *habit*. For them, smoking has become an unconscious act. They may light up or finish a smoke without being aware of it or taking much pleasure in it. The true habit smoker often doesn't enjoy smoking, but just buys and burns packs of cigarettes because he or she doesn't know what to do without them. Cutting down gradually may be quite effective if there is a change in the way cigarettes are smoked and the conditions under which they are smoked. They may not find it hard to quit once they make an effort to be conscious of each cigarette they smoke.

Finally, for some, smoking has become an *addiction*, a continual act of craving. These are the chain-smokers whose craving begins as soon as one cigarette is stubbed out. They may wake up in the morning and, despite a hacking cough, reach for a cigarette before they're out of bed. For these smokers, quitting is undoubtedly hard and must be generally done "cold turkey," since cutting down gradually is almost impossible. They must quit smoking as a conscious act of will, replacing the addiction to smoking with a turn toward health and self-control.

Since smoking depresses the appetite by dulling the senses of taste and smell, one of the immediate advantages of not smoking is being able to truly taste and smell food again. Because ex-smokers may satisfy their oral craving with food, and because of some other metabolic changes, many people gain weight when they quit. Weight gain can often be prevented by avoiding high-calorie foods, and by starting a moderate exercise program. People who have gained weight can generally return to their normal weight once they get used to their new and healthier lifestyle.

Helpful Tips for Quitting

• List your reasons for quitting. Concentrate on the reasons that are personally very important to you. Whenever you are tempted to smoke again, use the list to remind you about the unacceptable and unappetizing aspects of smoking.

• Emphasize the immediate benefits of quitting. If the long-term health benefits of quitting aren't sufficient motivation because they are too abstract or removed, concentrate on the immediate rewards of not smoking, such as cleaner breath, fresher clothes and hair, and improved stamina.

• Study your smoking habit. Keep a smoking diary to determine when and under what circumstances you smoke. The act of recording will help you become more conscious of your smoking.

• Plan your quitting. Set a date several weeks in advance and plan ahead. Some people are helped by tapering off smoking before the actual target date. Talk to friends who have quit and learn what to expect. Ask your doctor for advice.

• Let other people know you are quitting. This will help to initiate social support, and put social pressure on you to succeed. When someone offers you a cigarette, decline politely but firmly. Don't be afraid to ask others not to smoke in your presence.

Continued

• Try quitting with a friend, whenever possible. Keep in touch with one another on a daily basis.

• Examine your diet. Keep a food diary. Watch your weight. Eat small snacks, more frequently (five or six times a day), rather than three heavy meals. Keep a supply of low-calorie snacks on hand while reading or watching television. Avoid rich desserts, and eat fruits instead.

• The early period of quitting is not a good time for a stringent diet, since this may only lead to a return to the smoking habit.

• If you miss holding a cigarette, use substitutes such as pen or pencil, paper clip, or a key chain. If you miss the oral stimulation of a cigarette, use oral substitutes such as toothpicks, sugarless gum or candy, or a plastic straw.

• Increase your exercise. Regular exercise will help minimize the weight gain, will provide a sense of physical well-being, and will relieve "jittery nerves" and tension.

• Avoid situations in which you normally smoke. Avoid alcohol, coffee, or other beverages that you associate with smoking. Identify times when you are most likely to smoke, and plan other activities, such as taking a walk after dinner instead of having a second cup of coffee and a cigarette.

• Reward yourself! Begin putting away "cigarette money" to save for a trip, records, or new clothes. Or use the money periodically to buy a little something you wouldn't normally purchase, like a book, magazine, or fresh flowers.

4 Diet for a Healthy Heart

A large number of articles and books on dieting, often with conflicting advice, have been published in recent years. Unfortunately, a diet that is effective and appropriate for everyone does not exist. Studies have shown that modification of dietary habits, such as reducing the amount of fat and cholesterol in the diet, can lower the risk of coronary heart disease. Also, restriction of salt intake has been shown to be of benefit in patients with high blood pressure and in those with congestive heart failure.

A diet aimed at reducing the risk of heart disease should be directed primarily toward:

1) Reducing dietary fat and cholesterol
2) Increasing intake of complex carbohydrates
3) Achieving and maintaining a desirable body weight
4) Cutting down on salt intake

Reducing Dietary Fat and Cholesterol

Fats are complex molecules that are necessary for several essential body functions, such as storage of energy, support and protection of internal organs, and transportation of certain fat-soluble vitamins to the body tissues. Fats are popular constituents of our diet because they make foods taste better, providing flavor, aroma, and texture.

The fats in the bloodstream have two different origins: some come from the diet, and the rest are manufactured in the body (mostly inside the liver).

It should be noted that we do not need to eat any fat to acquire body fat; fat can be produced by the body from proteins and carbohydrates! In fact, that's exactly what happens if an individual consumes more calories than needed for his daily activities.

Depending on their chemical structure, fats are classified into two basic types: saturated and polyunsaturated (non-saturated). Saturated fats are found in foods of animal origin and dairy products, and in some vegetable oils (coconut and palm oils); they are generally solid at room temperature. Polyunsaturated fats are predominantly vegetable in origin, and are found in vegetable oils; they are usually liquid at room temperature.

Most vegetable oils containing polyunsaturated fats can be converted from their natural liquid form to become more solid and hardened. During the process, called hydrogenation, these oils become largely saturated, and thus resemble saturated fats. A certain amount of hydrogenation is needed to produce margarines which spread easily at room temperature.

Cholesterol is a fatty substance that is essential for certain bodily functions, such as the production of cell walls, hormones, and nerve function. Most of the cholesterol is manufactured in the body (primarily the liver), then sent through the bloodstream to cells throughout the body. The remainder of the cholesterol comes from the diet, almost exclusively from animal products. Even if the diet contained no cholesterol at all, the body would make enough of it out of other nutrients to satisfy all its needs. (For more information on cholesterol, see Chapter 2).

The level of cholesterol in the blood is influenced by the amount and kinds of fats we consume. Specifically, diets rich in saturated fats and cholesterol tend to raise the level of blood cholesterol, whereas diets rich in polyunsaturated fats help to keep it low. Monounsaturated fats appear to have no substantial effect on blood cholesterol level. Animal fats contain a high proportion of saturated fats, as well as cholesterol. Vegetable fats, on the other hand, contain mainly polyunsaturated fats, and no cholesterol.

The cholesterol level in the circulation can be lowered by making certain changes in the dietary fat intake, such as:

a) Reducing fat intake, especially saturated fats

b) Using polyunsaturated fats instead of saturated fats

c) Decreasing dietary cholesterol

a) Reducing Fat Intake, Especially Saturated Fats

Some of the foods containing a large amount of saturated fats include: red meat, sausages, whole milk, cream, butter, ice cream, cheese, hydrogenated margarines and shortenings, and bakery goods. These foods should be consumed only occasionally, or should be avoided altogether. Foods with lower fat content include: lean cuts of meat, chicken, fish, low-fat milk, skim-milk, and low-fat dairy products.

The current American diet contains about 40 percent of the total calories as fat. The recommended dietary goal is a diet that would contain less that 25 percent of total calories as fat. In order to achieve the desired reduction, it is not necessary to totally give up foods that contain fat. Instead, the reduction can be accomplished by making dietary adjustments: eating less of the foods with high fat content, and selecting foods with lower fat content to replace them.

b) Using Polyunsaturated Fats Instead of Saturated Fats

Polyunsaturated fats are commonly found in soft margarines, soft shortenings, and in vegetable oils (such as safflower, sunflower, corn, soybean, and cottonseed oils). Margarines vary considerably in their degree of saturation (or hydrogenation). In general, the more saturated a margarine is, the more solid it is at room temperature.

Polyunsaturated fats are recommended as a substitute for saturated fats, because they produce a cholesterol-lowering effect in the blood when included in the daily eating plan. It is not suggested, however, that people consume large quantities of polyunsaturated fats. They are certainly preferable to saturated fats, but there are good reasons to cut back on all fats. First, excessive fat intake of any kind contributes to weight gain and obesity. In addition, the effects of long-term consumption of large quantities of polyunsaturated fats are not known. In practical terms, it is recommended that people reduce saturated fats intake considerably, and use instead small amounts of the more polyunsaturated fats.

c) Decreasing Dietary Cholesterol

The cholesterol we consume is found exclusively in animal products. No cholesterol is found in foods of vegetable origin. Foods rich in cholesterol include egg yolks, red meats, organ meats (especially liver), and whole-milk dairy products. Contrary to what many people think, the cholesterol content of meat is associated primarily with the lean tissue, not the fat. In fact, equal weights of fatty and lean cuts of meat contain about equal amounts of cholesterol. Trimming meat is recommended not because it reduces cholesterol content but because it substantially reduces the saturated fat and calorie content.

The typical American diet supplies more than 500 milligrams of cholesterol a day over and above the amount of cholesterol made by the liver. The body's own cholesterol production decreases when cholesterol is eaten, but not enough to compensate for the amount consumed; blood cholesterol levels therefore rise. It is recommended that the average intake of cholesterol be reduced from the current 500 milligrams to less than 300 milligrams daily.

Helpful Tips: Eating Well the Low-Fat Way

• Limit meat consumption to one or two servings (3 to 6 ounces) per day. Fish and chicken contain less total fat and less saturated fat than red meat, and are therefore the preferred sources of animal protein.

• Choose lean cuts. Check meat for marbling (the white visible fat that runs through the red meat), and avoid well-marbled cuts.

• Trim off all visible fat before cooking your meat. The skin on chicken should be removed.

• Avoid meats with high-fat content, such as bacon, hamburgers, short ribs, frankfurters, luncheon meats, canned meat, and sausages.

• Broil, roast, or stir-fry meats, fish, and poultry rather than deep frying, sauteing, or stewing them.

• Make pot roasts and stews a day ahead. Chill them and scrape off fat that accumulates on top, then reheat.

• When sauteing or frying foods that don't need a lot of oil, brush the pan with oil just to coat it. Use a nonstick spray made from vegetable oil, or use a nonstick pan that requires no greasing.

Continued

• Switch to low-fat and skim milk dairy products. Use low-fat yogurt and ice milk in place of whole-milk yogurt and ice cream.

• Restrict your intake of hard and processed cheeses. They are high in fat and cholesterol. Use part-skimmed cheeses instead.

• When you cook, bake, or season your food, do not use saturated animal fats, such as butter or lard. Avoid solid vegetable shortenings. Instead, use polyunsaturated vegetable oils and margarine.

• Margarines vary considerably in their degree of saturation. As a general rule, the softer the margarine, the more unsaturated it is. Therefore, soft tubs margarines are preferred, because they are generally more unsaturated than stick margarines.

• When selecting a margarine, read the label. The first ingredient should be a "liquid vegetable oil." The phrase "partially hydrogenated" or "partially hardened" oil may appear among the ingredients, but should not be listed first.

• Be aware that when you see "contains no cholesterol" on a label you may still be getting a lot of fat in the product in the form of polyunsaturated or saturated vegetable fats!

• Limit your consumption of egg yolks to three a week, including those in prepared and processed foods (the yolk of a large egg contains 250 milligrams of cholesterol). Eggs whites contain no cholesterol and may be eaten freely.

• Limit your consumption of other cholesterol-rich foods, such as whole milk, whole-milk cheeses, whole-milk yogurt, sour cream, ice cream, butter, and organs meats (especially liver).

What about Fish Oils?

Until recently it was widely believed that consumption of fatty fish and shellfish should be avoided. Recent studies have shown, however, that the kind of fats found in fish and shellfish (unlike those found in red meat and poultry) are highly polyunsaturated. In fact, these marine fats, termed omega-3 fatty acids, have been found to be useful in lowering blood cholesterol levels, as well as making the platelets (the tiny blood cells involved in clotting) less sticky. It has been suggested that, by their actions, fish oils could actually prevent the buildup of fatty plaques and formation of blood clots inside the arteries. At this time, however, research is still at an early stage, and little is known about the actual benefits of fish oils in preventing coronary heart disease and strokes.

Press coverage of these recent studies has helped promote the use of fish-oil supplements. Capsules of fish oil containing a variety of marine fatty acids are now available in pharmacies and health-food stores. The usefulness and safety of these supplements have not been established, however, and their use remains experimental. For these reasons, most authorities in the field currently advise avoiding the consumption of fish-oil supplements, at least until further clinical trials become available. In the meantime, it is advisable to consume these oils by simply eating fish and shellfish; it is much more enjoyable, and there is still ample room for it as part of a well-balanced diet!

Increasing Intake of Complex Carbohydrates

All carbohydrates are made up of one or more molecules of sugar. Simple carbohydrates ("sugars"), are made of single or double molecules. Complex carbohydrates ("starches"), on the other hand, are made of branched chains of dozens of sugar molecules. All carbohydrates are readily broken down by the digestive enzymes into their component sugars and absorbed into the bloodstream. The liver converts all single molecules of sugar into glucose, commonly called "blood sugar." Glucose is the body's main energy source. It is the fuel the brain normally uses, and it is the main fuel for muscles. Without carbohydrates, the body would be forced to run on fat and proteins, a potentially dangerous situation.

Complex Carbohydrates Are "Good Food"

Complex carbohydrates are found in "starchy" foods such as potatoes, rice, corn, dried beans and peas, pasta, cereals, wheat, flour, and bread. They are also found in a variety of fresh fruits and vegetables. Foods high in complex carbohydrates are generally good sources of vitamins, minerals, and fiber, while being low in fat and devoid of cholesterol. These foods also make good low-cost substitutes for animal proteins.

Contrary to what many Americans think, complex carbohydrates are not "fattening." Ounce per ounce, they have the same number of calories as pure protein and less than half the calories of fat. If complex carbohydrates (like any other foods) are consumed in excess, however, they can contribute to weight gain.

The richest sources of vegetable protein are legumes, that is, peas and beans. All legumes can be a healthy substitute for animal protein in anyone's diet. Unlike proteins of animal source, proteins of vegetable origin are considered "incomplete." Therefore, in order to provide all the essential amino acids necessary for the body to manufacture protein from these carbohydrates, they should preferably be used in combinations, termed "complementary proteins." The amino acid balance of peas and beans, for example, can be improved by consuming them with grains (such as corn, rice, wheat, and barley).

Nuts (almonds, walnuts, pecans, cashews) and seeds (sesame, sun-flower) are also rich sources of vegetable protein. Unlike peas and beans, however, they contain too much fat to be used as a major source of protein on a regular basis. They are excellent as complements to other vegetable proteins, however.

Natural carbohydrate foods, particularly whole grains, beans, fresh fruits, and vegetables, are excellent sources of healthful dietary fiber. Fiber is a carbohydrate from plants that is not digested by the human digestive tract. It does supply "roughage," bulk that helps satisfy the appetite and keep the digestive system running smoothly.

About 45% of the total calories in the typical American diet are supplied by carbohydrates. Since the percentage of calories supplied by fats should decrease to 25% (from the current average of 40%), it is suggested that consumption of complex carbohydrates be increased to supply 60% of the calories in a typical diet (see figure 5).

What About Sugar?

Today, a major portion of carbohydrates in the American diet comes from refined or processed sugars, which are extracted from their natural sources and added to foods that do not naturally contain them. Many Americans consume over 500 calories of sugar and other sweeteners a day,

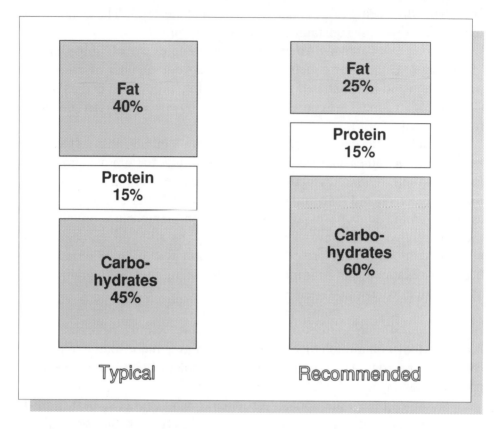

Figure 5. The fat, protein, and carbohydrate content of the typical American diet, and the recommended diet (as percent of calories).

primarily from soft drinks, desserts, candy, jelly, and syrup. Many packaged foods are high in sugar, often adding calories without providing other essential nutrients.

There is little question that sugar in the diet promotes tooth decay. Sugar is also fattening; a lot of sugar calories can get packed into a rather small quantity of food. By eating sweets, people are more likely to overconsume calories long before the stomach is full, thus overloading the body with calories.

For these reasons, it is suggested that sweets be eaten only occasionally, rather than as part of the daily diet. It is recommended that the portion of calories derived from refined and processed sugar drop from the current 20 percent down to 10 percent or less. The major portion of carbohydrates should be in the form of complex carbohydrates ("starchy" foods) and naturally occurring sugars found in fresh fruits and vegetables.

Achieving and Maintaining a Desirable Body Weight

The management of obesity poses a difficult challenge. Studies have shown that although obesity is preventable, it is almost never "curable." Regardless of the weight reduction method used, most people will fail to lose weight or maintain the weight loss for any significant length of time. "Fad" diets, which are practically a way of life for millions of Americans, may help to shed pounds fast, but those pounds rarely stay off.

The difficulties in weight reduction have helped popularize a number of diets based on the premise that weight can be lost by changing the composition of the diet without reducing the quantity of calories consumed. Diets such as the high protein, high fat, or low carbohydrate plans are some of the most popular. The evidence shows, however, that these diets may have serious side effects and that weight is often regained rapidly once the diet is over.

The basic principle of weight gain is simple: people gain weight because they consume more calories (whether from carbohydrate, protein, or fat) than they use. Most authorities on the subject agree that the only reliable way to lose weight is by creating a negative caloric balance, that is, expending more calories than are being consumed. This can be achieved through reduction of caloric intake or through increase of caloric expenditure, or a combination of both. In simpler words, the answer to the problem of obesity is to eat less, eat properly, and exercise more!

As a rule of thumb, a change in food intake equivalent to 3500 calories will result in a weight loss of 1 pound. Thus, by consuming 500 fewer calories a day, dieters can lose 1 pound per week. They can do the same by burning up 500 calories per day through exercise.

If weight loss is necessary, a sensible approach and a moderate loss of about 2 pounds per week is recommended. A slow and steady approach, using a balanced combination of essential nutrients, is the only safe method of weight loss. "Fad" diets that emphasize one category of food and promise rapid weight loss can cause a chemical imbalance in the body and result in dangerous medical conditions. For the individual who is severely obese and must lose a large amount of weight rapidly, it is imperative to have a complete medical evaluation and to diet under the supervision of a physician.

Whether the individual follows a diet prescribed by a physician, a nutritionist, or a weight-reduction group is a matter of personal choice. Some dieters may find it easier to diet with a group, which often helps to boost motivation by providing peer support. Weight reduction programs (such as Weight Watchers®) offer sensible, well-balanced diet plans, plus plenty of tips and moral support from group leaders and members.

Helpful Tips: Keeping Those Extra Pounds Off

• Plan a well-balanced diet around familiar foods. Choose lower calorie foods and lower calorie ways of food preparation. Include fresh vegetables and fruits at every meal because they are low in calories and high in bulk.

• Learn the amount of calories in foods you eat. Study a comprehensive calorie chart to familiarize yourself with foods that are unexpectedly rich in calories. Learn to judge portions accurately.

• Try to eat three meals a day at fairly regular times. Eat only at the kitchen table or dining-room table, at a place that has been set with silverware and a plate.

• Don't skip meals. It will lower your resistance to snacking between meals. You may end up consuming more calories than if you had eaten a real meal.

• Eat sensible portions. Don't eat "family style." When you put your portion on a plate, do it away from the table.

• Learn to stop eating before you feel "full." The slight hunger you may feel will disappear about a half hour after meal time.

Continued

• Don't watch television or read while you eat. Instead, concentrate on your meal. This will make the meal more satisfying and will help you eat less.

• Budget your calories to take care of snacks, weekend eating, and holidays. Plan ahead for special occasions by eating less at breakfast and lunch.

• Don't keep high-calorie snack foods around. Stock up on low-calorie substitutes. Cut up a bag full of fresh vegetables or a bowl of fresh fruit and set it aside, ready for consumption.

• Go grocery shopping after you've eaten a satisfying meal. Do not buy foods that are likely to be tempting or high in calories.

• Let your family and friends know that you're trying to cut down. Ask them to help by not tempting you with foods you love.

• When eating out, practice portion control. Most restaurants give servings that are far larger than you would dish up for yourself at home. You don't have to finish it all. Offer some to a tablemate or take home a "doggie bag."

• Avoid fast food restaurants. Fast foods, such as hamburgers and French fries, are loaded with fat (mostly saturated), calories, and salt.

• Limit your alcohol consumption, and stay away form high-calorie mixers and sweet liqueurs. Ounce per ounce, alcohol has nearly as many calories as fat. When you're ready for a refill, try plain soda or mineral water with a wedge of lemon or lime.

• A sensible program of regular exercise, preferably every day, should become an integral part of your weight-control program.

• Make exercise part of your daily activities. Walk whenever possible. Use the stairs for a few flights instead of taking the elevator.

• Don't let an occasional indulgence be an excuse for going completely "overboard." If you have "blown" your diet, you can make up for it by cutting back a little the next day, or by getting some extra exercise.

As we have seen, it is important to increase caloric expenditure in order to burn excess body fat. This can be achieved by regular exercise activity. There is no need to start a strenuous exercise program or to become an "exercise nut" to put activity back into one's life. Energy can be spent by integrating some physical activity during the course of a day, such as walking instead of riding, and climbing a few flights of stairs instead of taking the elevator.

Without changing behavior at the same time, however, the dropout rate in weight reduction programs is discouragingly high, as are the chances of gaining the weight back. Behavior modification is a method that deals directly with the underlying cause of obesity, namely, the eating behavior. It focuses on changing eating habits so that weight loss may be maintained on a long-term basis. Behavior modification does not promise a shortcut to successful weight loss, and it is neither quick nor especially easy. It rather emphasizes gradual weight loss, and provides new eating habits that will help maintain the loss.

Cutting Down on Salt

Salt is made up of sodium and chloride, two minerals that are essential in the maintenance of the body's fluid balance. The salt-fluid balance is controlled to a large degree by the kidneys. If an excessive amount of salt is ingested, the kidneys may not be able to excrete the salt load, and as a result, the volume of fluid in the body gradually increases.

Salt, when consumed in excessive amount, may cause an elevation of the blood pressure in susceptible people. Studies have shown, for example, that adding salt to foods or eating foods high in salt are the factors that most likely contribute to the age-related tendency to develop hypertension. In patients with impaired cardiac function, excessive salt intake may lead to accumulation of extra fluid in the body tissues, and thus to worsening of symptoms of congestive heart failure.

Most Americans consume more salt than their bodies need. After sugar, salt is our leading food additive, in foods prepared out and at home. The average American consumes 10 to 15 grams of salt daily, the equivalent of 4 to 6 grams of sodium a day (1 gram of salt contains 400 milligrams, or 0.4 grams, of sodium). The body's actual physiological requirements are probably below 400 milligrams of sodium a day. To be on the safe side, the recommended daily allowance (RDA) for adults is 1,200 to 3,600 milligrams of sodium, or 3 to 8 grams of salt per day (one teaspoon is about 5 grams salt).

When adding up the amount of salt we eat, it is not enough to count only what is added to foods when cooking them or at the table. Some sources of salt are obvious, such as salted crackers, nuts, pretzels, potato chips, pickles, herring, soy sauce and sauerkraut. Other sources of salt, however, are less obvious or "hidden." Some of the sodium in our diet, for example, is already in the food as it comes from the earth (spinach, celery, beets) and animal (meat, dairy products). Drinking water may also be an important hidden source of sodium.

The major hidden source of salt, however, comes from processed foods (which today account for over half of the food Americans eat). Salt and other sodium compounds are added to foods not only to make them taste better but also to improve color and texture and to preserve them. Among the processed foods containing a high level of sodium are: cheese, cereals, bread, luncheon meats, pudding, baked goods, pancakes, soups, and canned vegetables. These products are heavily laced with salt as well as other sources of sodium, such as leavening agents, baking powder, baking soda, and a variety of other food additives. Another hidden source of sodium is medications, particularly some over-the-counter medicines.

Although the precise health benefits of salt restriction in a healthy person are yet to be proved, it is reasonable to recommend moderation in salt intake. By simply avoiding foods that are high in sodium, and by not using the salt shaker at the table, most people can markedly reduce their overall salt intake. This reduction of salt intake is likely to reduce the risk of high blood pressure in susceptible persons. Furthermore, consuming less salt has not been shown to harm anyone.

Sodium restriction is generally recommended in patients with high blood pressure and in those with congestive heart failure. The desired degree of sodium restriction can be usually accomplished by having the patient follow several simple guidelines, such as: a) not adding salt to food during cooking or at the table; b) avoiding obviously salty foods such as pickles, salted peanuts, and potato chips; c) avoiding or minimizing the use of canned or prepacked foods; and d) recognizing the salt content of various foods by reading the package labels.

Helpful Tips: Shaking the Salt Habit

• Start by not adding salt at the table, and certainly never add salt before you have tasted the food.

• Eat only limited amounts, or avoid altogether, foods high in sodium such as: luncheon meats (salami, bologna), smoked meats (ham, bacon, sausage, corned beef), canned foods that list salt on their labels, packaged bouillon, and certain condiments (catsup, chili sauce, mustard, and barbecue sauce).

• Gradually reduce the amount of salt you use in cooking and baking. As you get used to less and less salt, you will find you need to add only a fraction of the original amount.

• Experiments with seasonings, herbs, and spices, using them in place of salt. Examples: onions, garlic, pepper, dry mustard, lemon juice.

• Clearly, the best way to avoid salt is to buy and cook as many fresh foods as possible.

• If you are on a sodium-restricted diet, check the label on all processed foods for sodium content. If you are dependent on processed foods, look for those labeled "low sodium" or "low salt."

• Unless advised by your physician, try to avoid using salt substitutes in which all or part of the sodium has been replaced with potassium.

• If you are on sodium restricted diet, check with your doctor before taking antacids, cough preparations, and laxatives. Many of these items contain significant amount of sodium.

Although the sodium in the diet could be restricted to as low as 400 milligrams per day, the development of effective diuretic drugs and the difficulty in following a severely sodium restricted diet have made the use of such diets less desirable. The most common sodium-restricted diets are the "Low-salt Diet," which contains about 3 grams sodium, and the "2-gram Sodium Diet." On the "Low-salt Diet," food can be salted in ordinary amounts during cooking, but the use of highly salted foods and the addition of salt at the table are eliminated.

Salt substitutes can be used to add a salt-like flavor to foods. The main ingredient of most salt substitutes is potassium chloride, which may be harmful to some people. Patients should therefore check with their physician before using them. This applies to low-sodium meat tenderizers and seasoned salt substitutes as well.

Guidelines: The Balanced Diet

• Variety in the diet is necessary if you want to obtain the proper balance of needed nutrients (proteins, carbohydrates, fats, minerals, vitamins, fiber, etc.). Besides, a varied diet is more interesting than a "boring" one. There are dozens of tasty new ways to combine familiar ingredients that you may have never thought of before.

• Start thinking about how to make sensible selections within the framework of the basic food groups:

a) *Bread, cereals, pasta, legumes, and grains:* These foods are rich in complex carbohydrates, vitamins, and fiber. They are low in fat and contain no cholesterol. Combinations of legumes (dry beans and peas) with grains (corn, rice, wheat, barley) can be used as substitutes for animal protein.

b) *Fruits and vegetables:* They are rich in complex carbohydrates, natural sugars, fiber, minerals, and vitamins. They are low in fat, calories, and sodium. They contain no cholesterol. The most nutritious way to eat fruits and vegetables is raw.

c) *Milk and dairy products:* These foods are good sources of protein, vitamins, and minerals. They contain fat as well. Low-fat milk and dairy products are preferable to whole-milk products.

d) *Meat, poultry, fish, and eggs:* These foods are rich in protein, vitamins, and minerals. Unfortunately, they are also rich in fat, cholesterol, and calories. They should be consumed in moderation (3 to 6 oz. a day). Fish and poultry (without the skin) are the preferable sources in this group.

e) *Vegetable fats and oils:* Should be used in small amounts.

Continued

• In each food category, choose those foods that are lower in fat, especially in saturated fats, lower in cholesterol, lower in added sweeteners, and lower in sodium.

• Moderation in your eating habits is important. Unless you have a specific health problem that requires you to steer clear of certain foods, there is no reason why you should totally give up foods you especially enjoy. It's often a question of tradeoffs. If you eat a high-fat food for breakfast, for example, choose those low in fat for the rest of your meals that day.

• Changes in the diet should be gradual. If changes are too abrupt, you are likely to resent them and will probably build up cravings for favorite foods you have excluded from the menu.

For Further Reading

Jane Brody, *Jane Brody's Nutrition Book: A Lifetime Guide to Good Eating for Better Health and Weight Control.* New York: Norton, 1981.

Jane Brody, *Jane Brody's Good Food Book: Living the High-Carbohydrate Way.* New York: Norton, 1985.

Sonja L. Connor, and William E. Connor, *The New American Diet.* New York: Simon and Schuster, 1986.

Michael E. DeBakey, et al., *The Living Heart Diet.* New York: Simon and Schuster, 1984.

5 Exercise and Cardiovascular Fitness

Although many more Americans are now involved in regular exercise then ever before, most still do not get enough physical activity. In today's society, the expanded use of mechanical energy to replace human physical energy encourages a sedentary lifestyle. Most Americans drive to work and to stores, use elevators instead of stairs, become spectators rather than participants at sports, and do little heavy labor on their jobs.

Regular exercise activity has been shown to reduce the risk of coronary heart disease (see page 18). It also has a positive effect on other risk factors; regular exercise tends to lower blood pressure, helps control weight, and increases the blood level of HDL cholesterol (the "good" cholesterol). In addition, many smokers give up the habit once they start exercising.

Cardiovascular fitness is an observable and predictable benefit of exercise training. It is a state of body efficiency that enables a person to exercise for longer periods of time without excessive fatigue, and to respond to sudden physical demands with an economy of heartbeats and only a modest rise in blood pressure. The physically fit individual is able to supply more energy to his muscles so that they can work harder and longer, and with less effort.

Besides lowering the risk of heart disease and improving cardiovascular fitness, exercise provides several other benefits. Exercise activity enhances a person's sense of well-being; it helps release tension, and it promotes relaxation and better sleep. Regular exercise helps in coping with stress, anxiety, and depression. People who exercise regularly tend to be more energetic, enthusiastic, and optimistic. In addition to benefitting the cardiovascular system, regular exercise improves muscle tone and flexibility, and helps lose those extra pounds.

Before Starting an Exercise Program

Any person starting an exercise program, especially someone who has been sedentary, should not try to do too much, too soon. Going "all out" from the start could be the quickest way to cool one's resolve! Any exercise program should start at a low level of intensity and then progress gradually and sensibly over a period of time. After being accustomed to a certain level of exercise, the individual will then be prepared for more demanding activities.

It is probably true that most individuals would have no problem engaging in a gradual and sensible exercise program. For some people, however, exercise can be dangerous. As many as 10 percent of apparently normal adults over the age of 40 may have hidden heart disease or disorders of the musculoskeletal (pertaining to muscles and bones) system. It is therefore recommended that all persons over the age 40, especially those who are not accustomed to vigorous exercise, consult their physician and undergo a medical checkup prior to starting an exercise program. Individuals with a history of heart disease or cardiac symptoms, those with one or more major risk factors, and those with a family history of premature heart disease should be screened, even if younger than 40.

The medical checkup will focus on the cardiovascular system. The physician will inquire about the presence of any cardiac symptoms (such as chest pain, shortness of breath, or palpitations), history of heart problems, the presence of major risk factors for coronary heart disease (such as smoking, elevated blood cholesterol, high blood pressure), and family history of premature heart disease. He will then measure the blood pressure, and perform a thorough examination of the heart and blood vessels. Finally, he will carefully examine the bones, joints and muscles, looking for the presence of any abnormalities. Basic laboratory tests generally include blood tests (analyzed for cholesterol, potassium, glucose, etc.), and an electrocardiogram (ECG).

Depending on the data obtained during the medical checkup the physician may recommend an exercise stress test ("treadmill"). During the test, the individual walks on a motor driven treadmill (or in some cases rides a stationary bicycle) while his heartbeat, ECG, and blood pressure are being monitored. The stress test measures the performance of the cardiovascular system during exercise. This "road test" is used primarily as a diagnostic tool to uncover the presence of hidden heart problems before the unwary exerciser begins the program. It is also used to assess the individual's level of cardiovascular fitness in order to design a personalized fitness program. The existence of heart disease and impaired heart function would not necessarily preclude an exercise program. In fact, if prescribed appropriately, exercise may actually improve the condition.

Important!

Prior to starting an exercise program, you should consult a doctor if any one or more of the following apply to you:

• You are over 40 and not accustomed to vigorous exercise.

• You have a history of a heart problem (such as angina, heart attack, heart murmur, cardiac arrhythmias, etc.).

• You tend to develop exercise-related symptoms (such as chest pain, arm pain, extreme breathlessness, faintness, etc.).

• You smoke; have high blood pressure; or have a high blood level of cholesterol.

• You are 20 lbs. or more overweight.

• You have a family history of premature heart disease.

• You suffer from a medical condition which may require special medical attention during an exercise program (such as joint or bone problems, insulin-dependent diabetes, etc.).

The Ingredients of a Good Exercise Program

When designing an exercise program, the key ingredients for such a program include:

• the type of physical activity
• the intensity, duration, and frequency of the exercise
• the warm-up and cool-down periods

Type of Physical Activity

Not all types of exercise are equally useful for promoting cardiovascular fitness. Only those exercises which significantly increase the continuous flow of blood through the heart, lungs, and large skeletal muscles are beneficial. These exercises are termed "dynamic." Walking, jogging, swimming, and bicycling, for example, require continuous movement of the legs and arms. This results in rhythmic tensing and relaxing of muscles, and thus helps the flow of blood. On the other hand, some types of exercise, such as weight lifting, cause the muscles being strengthened to contract and tense up. The pressure squeezes the blood vessels, letting less blood pass instead of more.

Certain kinds of exercise may enhance blood flow but still do not improve cardiovascular fitness, because they cannot be kept up for a sufficiently long period of time. Thus, the second requirement for the right type of exercise is that it must be capable of being sustained; it must be *aerobic* (meaning "with oxygen"). An aerobic exercise is the type which steadily supplies enough oxygen to the exercising muscles for as long as the exercise is continued.

Any rhythmic, repetitive, dynamic activity which can be continued for two or more minutes, without gasping for air afterwards, is probably aerobic. Sprinting, for example, is not an aerobic exercise (it is anaerobic); the sprinter can't keep going at that pace for too long. By contrast, the experienced jogger can cover long distances almost effortlessly, because his body has attained a balance between the oxygen it needs and the oxygen it is getting through the lungs and cardiovascular system.

Good aerobic exercises include brisk walking, jogging, running, bicycling, swimming, cross-country skiing, skating, tennis (singles), dancing, "aerobics" workouts, and jumping rope. Exercises which are not considered aerobic include bowling, golf, weight lifting, down-hill skiing, tennis (doubles), baseball, and volleyball. Although some of these exercises may seem strenuous, the level of activity is usually not sustained long enough to be aerobic; they do not improve endurance or "wind." Of course, types of exercise which do not improve cardiovascular fitness may have other benefits, such as gaining muscle strength, increasing body flexibility, and improving athletic skills.

Intensity, Duration, and Frequency

Cardiovascular conditioning occurs when a particular program involves an aerobic activity performed:

- at an intensity level within the "target zone"
- for a duration of 20 to 30 minutes per session
- at a frequency of 3 to 4 times a week.

The maximum heart rate is the highest level an individual's pulse rate can reach. It can be estimated by subtracting the person's age from 220. Exercise below 60 percent of the maximum heart rate gives the heart and lungs little if any conditioning effect. Anything above 85 percent, on the other hand, adds little benefit for a great deal of extra exercise, and can be potentially dangerous. The area between these two heart rates is known as the "target zone," the goal for which an individual should strive in order to improve cardiovascular fitness (see figure 6). The ideal training goal is generally around the 75 percent level.

The numerical values for the maximum heart rate and the target zone are only "average" values based on the person's age. As many as one third of the population may differ from these values. For example, a normal 60-year-old person may have a higher than normal maximum heart rate of 180. A 30-year-old individual, on the other hand, may have a maximum heart rate of only 170.

Exercisers should be aware that some medications and medical conditions can affect the maximum heart rate and the target zone values. The beta blockers (drugs taken for the treatment of high blood pressure and angina), for example, may slow the pulse rate and thus lower the target zone. Therefore, anyone taking cardiovascular drugs should consult his physician to determine whether the heart rate values should be adjusted.

Individuals can determine if they are within their target zone by taking their pulse immediately after the exercise activity. The easiest way to do this is to place 2 or 3 fingers lightly over the carotid artery (located on either side of the Adam's Apple), count the pulse for 10 seconds, and then multiply that number by 6 (thus giving the pulse rate per minute). Another convenient spot for checking the pulse is at the wrist, just below the base of the thumb. The exercise pulse rate should be checked about once a week during the first 3 months of exercising, and periodically thereafter.

Age	Target Zone, 60-85% (beats per minute)	Average Maximum Heart Rate (100%)
20	120 - 170	200
25	117 - 166	195
30	114 - 162	190
35	111 - 157	185
40	108 - 153	180
45	105 - 149	175
50	102 - 145	170
55	99 - 140	165
60	96 - 136	160
65	93 - 132	155
70	90 - 128	150

Figure 6. The target zone heart rates, according to age.

At the beginning of the program, an individual should exercise at a level of 60 percent of the maximum heart rate, and then gradually increase the intensity, over a period of weeks or months. For those who have been sedentary for years, it may be wise to wait several months before raising the heart rate above the 70 percent level.

In order to provide a conditioning effect, the exercise session should last 20 to 30 minutes. For beginners who are out of shape and may have trouble sustaining exercise at target zone intensity for that long, the duration of exercise can be adjusted. They can begin exercising at a target zone intensity for only 5 or 10 minutes a session, then gradually build up duration. Alternating exercise of high intensity and low intensity (such as jogging and walking) is another way to start.

For those beginning an exercise program, the optimal frequency for exercise is 3 or 4 times a week, on nonconsecutive days. Although the "training effect" on the body increases somewhat if the exercise is done more frequently, so does the chance of joint and muscle injury, particularly with exercises like jogging and running. For those who walk or swim (where the risk of injury is small), and those who exercise for weight control, the frequency can be increased, up to a daily schedule.

As the individual continues to exercise and the heart becomes better conditioned, either the intensity or the duration will have to be increased, in order to maintain the training effect. A bicycle rider, for example, should either have to pedal longer, pedal faster, or begin cycling up hills or in a lower gear to increase the resistance.

Warm-up and Cool-down Periods

Often overlooked is the importance of the warm-up and cool-down periods. The *warm-up period* helps stretch and loosen up the body muscles. It also stimulates the circulation, increases the heart rate, and prepares the cardiovascular system for the aerobic phase of the exercise session. A 5-minute warming up period will reduce the risk of muscle or joint injury, and will prevent the risk of abruptly overtaxing the cardiovascular system. The warm-up should begin with undemanding exercises, such as swinging the arms, and gently stretching the back, neck, and legs. Emphasis should be given to stretching the backs of the legs (hamstring and calf muscles). The warm-up may then become more dynamic, perhaps with slow walking, jumping jacks, or running in place.

Equally important is the *cool-down period*. During a vigorous workout, blood vessels in the extremities become dilated, so that they can supply additional blood and oxygen to the exercising muscles. The pumping action of the contracting muscles helps return blood toward the heart. If one abruptly stops exercising, the pumping action of the skeletal muscles stops. The blood vessels, however, remain dilated. This may result in "pooling" of blood in the extremities, reduction of blood return to the heart, and a drop in the amount of blood pumped by the heart. This explains why abrupt stopping of vigorous exercise can result in dizziness and even fainting. A 5-minute cooling down period allows a gradual slowing of the heart rate and a safer recovery. The cool-down exercises generally consist of a brief relaxed walk and some stretching of the body and extremities.

Selecting an Exercise Program

When selecting a specific exercise program, several factors should be considered, such as: the health and physical capabilities of the individual; the equipment and facilities required; the weather and seasonal variability; the person's schedule; and last but not least, the individual's interests and preferences.

The aerobic activity chosen should provide enough exercise to get the body functioning at the target heart rate for a period of at least 20 to 30 minutes per session. It should be demanding but not exhausting, and need not become competitive. The type of exercise should provide some pleasure and enjoyment; it should be an activity that interests the person enough to motivate him to continue with it for an indefinite number of years.

Brisk *walking* is by far the most convenient form of exercise. This enjoyable activity can be performed almost anywhere; it is the easiest to fit into a hectic daily routine; it can easily be done alone or in a group; and it requires no athletic skill or talent. It is also the easiest to monitor with respect to pulse rates, time, and distance. Walking appeals particularly to people for whom more strenuous activities are either unappealing or medically ill-advised. Walking is great for confirmed nonathletes, overweight people, and those suffering from heart disease, chronic lung disease, and arthritis.

Jogging and *running* offer the most intense aerobic workout in the shortest amount of time, and provide an efficient way for getting lower-body muscular conditioning. Jogging is popular because it can be done almost anywhere, and requires no special equipment other than comfortable shoes. Jogging is recommended for people with healthy knees and feet. People who do not warm up properly and those who begin to run excessive distances are at higher risk of sustaining muscle and joint injuries. It is best to start with the walking program for several weeks, then progressively ease into the jogging program, by alternating periods of walking and jogging within the same exercise session.

Swimming involves all of the major muscles in the body and it therefore gives more of a total conditioning effect than many other sports. It is a convenient activity if one has access to a swimming pool. Just paddling about or floating in the water, however, is not adequate for cardiovascular conditioning! The real benefit of swimming will come only when one is able to swim lap after lap effortlessly for 20 minutes or more. Swimming is an excellent activity for obese individuals and for those who have leg joint problems or who have sustained injuries in other sports.

Bicycling appeals to a lot of people because it is more fun than walking or jogging. Bicycling, though, is not as aerobic as jogging or running. It is almost exclusively a lower-body activity, and thus helpful in the conditioning of the leg muscles. Like swimming, it is a non-weight bearing activity, and is therefore a terrific choice for anyone with chronic joint or foot problems. There is relatively little danger of serious muscle and joint injury (injuries may result, however, from accidental encounters with the road, motorists, or other cyclists). Stationary bicycles provide the convenience of use at home, even during poor weather. Most modern stationary bicycles are equipped with a speedometer and with resistance controls, allowing easy monitoring of the exercise workload.

"Aerobics" workouts have become very popular in the past decade or two. It is one of the more enjoyable and exciting activities, combining exercise, dance steps, and disco music. It can be performed either in large groups or in the privacy of one's home. It can be done at the person's own pace. To be effective, the exercise should be performed at an intensity level that raises the heartbeat to within the target heart rate, and for at least 20 minutes. For the beginner, exercise classes lasting 30 to 45 minutes, with ample time for warm-up and cool-down periods, are recommended.

· · · · · ·

The various types of aerobic exercise are not equal in their capacity to induce cardiovascular fitness. The number of calories expended varies with the activity in question. (See figure 7).

Following are a few examples of caloric expenditures for selected physical activities, based on an average body size of 150 lbs. (values are higher for larger persons):

Type of activity	Cals. per hour
Walking, 2 to 4 mph	200 - 400
Jogging, 5 to 7 mph	500 - 800
Running, 8 to 10 mph	900 - 1200
Cycling, 6 mph	250 - 300
Cycling, 12 mph	400 - 500
Swimming, breaststroke	300 - 600
Swimming, crawl	600 - 900
Aerobics workout	300 - 500
Tennis, singles	400 - 500

Figure 7. Calorie expenditure for selected physical activities.

The Risks of Exercise

Exercise in most of its forms can be associated with a certain degree of risk. The potential risks may include:

a) Muscle and joint injuries: This is the most common problem associated with exercise. The injuries most frequently result from exercising too hard or for too long, particularly in persons who have been sedentary for some time.

b) Heat exhaustion and heat stroke: These are relatively rare problems. They generally occur during hot and humid days, if proper precautions are not taken. Symptoms of heat exhaustion may include intense thirst, weakness, lightheadedness, headache, nausea, and confusion. Heat stroke is characterized, in addition, by dangerous elevation of body temperature, dry skin (sweating stops), and loss of consciousness. Heat stroke is a medical emergency.

c) Motor vehicles injuries: They may occur if the exerciser is struck by a car while jogging or bicycling. They may result in major injury.

d) Major cardiac events: On rare occasion, strenuous exercise activity can result in a heart attack or sudden death.

So, Is It Safe to Exercise?

In view of these potential risks of exercising, particularly the possibility of sustaining a heart attack or sudden death, one may wonder whether vigorous exercise is really safe. Before attempting to answer this important question, several comments should be made:

First of all, the actual risk of suffering a massive heart attack or dying as a result of vigorous exercise is very small. Out of hundreds of thousands of people who exercise each day, the reported cases of sudden death are extremely rare.

Second, the cardiac event is not necessarily the result of the exercise activity itself, but may rather be coincidental. In fact, the vast majority of fatal cardiac events occur under resting conditions (such as sitting, driving, watching TV, sleeping, etc.) and not during physical activity!

Third, the majority of individuals who suffer a cardiac event during exercise do have severe underlying heart disease. In persons over 40, the most common underlying condition is coronary heart disease, that is, severe narrowing of the coronary arteries.

Finally, in many of these individuals, the cardiac event is preceded by cardiac symptoms (such as chest pain, severe breathlessness, and faintness), but for some reason these warning signs are either ignored or denied!

Based on these facts, it appears that exercise is indeed safe, provided that certain precautions are taken. Furthermore, considering all the benefits exercise can bring, one should wonder whether it is safe not to exercise!

Guidelines: Precautions for Safe Exercise

Many exercise-related risks and injuries can be prevented by taking proper precautions. Here are some guidelines:

• Set realistic goals! Don't push yourself into doing too much too soon. Start slowly and increase speed, distance, and duration gradually. An optimal training goal is 75 percent of your maximum heart rate.

• Listen to your body! If you develop muscle and joint pains, you are probably progressing too fast. Don't make the mistake of exercising beyond these early warning signs, since more serious injuries may result.

• Warm up thoroughly prior to the workout, to stretch the muscles and tendons, and to stimulate the circulation.

• Cool down properly following the workout, to allow the body to recover gradually.

• Stop exercising if you feel lightheaded, breathless, nauseated, or overly tired.

• Stop exercising and call your doctor if, during or following exercise, you develop pain in your chest or arms, cold sweat, extreme breathless-ness, palpitations, or faintness.

• Use proper clothing. Don't overdress for exercise in warm or hot weather. Use proper equipment and facilities.

• Drink water before and after exercising, especially on a hot day. Avoid exercise on very hot and humid days (when the temperature is above 90° F, or the humidity above 80 percent).

• Wait at least 2 hours after a heavy meal before exercising, and at least 4 hours after consuming alcohol.

• Finally, take proper precautions to avoid automobile injuries: If walking or jogging in the dark (or when it's not fully light), wear light-colored clothes or a reflecting band, so that drivers can see you. Face oncoming traffic.

Part Two

DIAGNOSING
HEART DISEASE

6 The Heart: A Magnificent Pump

The heart is a muscular hollow organ that pumps a continuous flow of blood throughout the circulatory system. It lies in the middle of the chest, slightly to the left, and is protected by the sternum (breastbone) and the rib cage (see figure 8). It is about the size of one's clenched fist, and weighs less than a pound. The heart is one of nature's most efficient and durable pumps. Each day it beats more than 100,000 times, and each day it pumps nearly 2000 gallons of blood! The heart works day and night, every day of one's life, resting only in between beats, for a split-second pause.

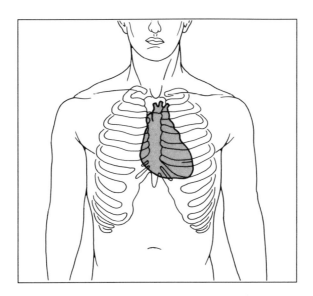

Figure 8. The position of the heart, behind the breastbone and rib cage.

How the Heart Works

The heart is made of muscle tissue called myocardium (or heart muscle). It is divided into a "left side" and a "right side" by a solid wall of muscle, termed the septum. (See figure 9). On each side of the septum there are two *chambers:* an upper chamber, or atrium, which receives blood from the veins and acts as a reservoir; and a lower chamber, or ventricle, which functions as a pumping chamber, after having received blood from the atrium. The left ventricle is the main pumping chamber, pumping blood under high pressure to all parts of the body, except the lungs. The right ventricle, which has thinner walls, sends blood only to the lungs.

To regulate the flow of blood within the heart there are four *valves,* which function like one-way doors, allowing the blood to circulate in only one direction, and preventing it from backing up. The valves are ringlike structures with two or three tissue flaps, called cusps or leaflets, that open and close depending upon the force of blood within the heart chambers. On the left side of the heart there are two valves: the mitral valve, located between the left atrium and the left ventricle, and the aortic valve, located between the left ventricle and the aorta (the body's main artery). The corresponding valves on the right side of the heart are the tricuspid valve, located between the right atrium and the right ventricle, and the pulmonic valve, located between the right ventricle and the pulmonary artery.

As it beats, the heart pumps blood through a system of *blood vessels,* elastic-like tubes that carry blood to every part of the body. Blood leaves the heart in arteries and returns to it in veins. The body's main artery, the aorta, is about an inch wide, and it divides into several large arteries conducting blood to the different parts of the body. The large arteries branch off like a tree into smaller and smaller arteries, and finally divide into tiny blood vessels, the capillaries, which link the arteries to the veins. The capillaries deliver oxygen and other nutrients through their thin walls directly to the cells around them, and at the same time they pick up carbon dioxide and other waste products from the cells. From the smallest veins, the oxygen-depleted blood passes into larger and larger veins and returns back to the heart. The vast network of blood vessels including arteries, capillaries and veins is over 60,000 miles long, which is more than twice the distance around the world!

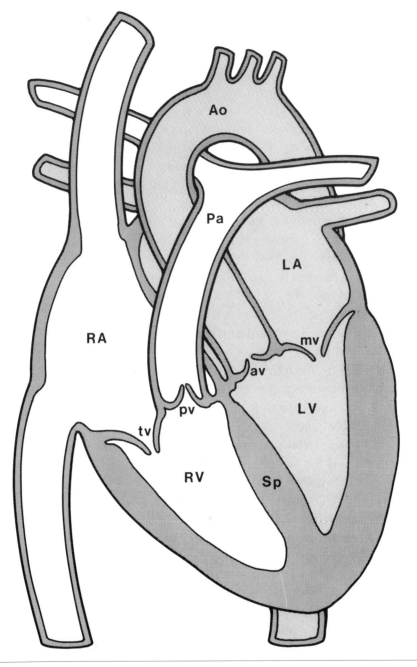

LA - Left atrium	mv - mitral valve	Sp - Septum
LV - Left ventricle	av - aortic valve	Ao - Aorta
RA - Right atrium	tv - tricuspid valve	Pa - Pulmonary
RV - Right ventricle	pv - pulmonic valve	artery

Figure 9. The heart chambers, heart valves, and major blood vessels.

There is a continuous flow of blood throughout the *circulatory system.* (See figure 10). The oxygen-poor blood coming from the body collects in the right atrium and then flows into the right ventricle through the tricuspid valve. As the right ventricle contracts it pumps blood through the pulmonic valve into the pulmonary arteries and to the lungs. Within the lungs, as we breathe, the carbon dioxide is released and fresh oxygen is picked up.

The oxygen-rich blood then flows into the left atrium, and into the left ventricle across the mitral valve. The left ventricle is the main pumping chamber and therefore the more muscular one. As it contracts, blood is pumped under high pressure across the aortic valve into the aorta. The oxygen-rich blood is carried through large arteries, smaller arteries, and capillaries, and reaches millions of cells in the different organs and tissues. It then flows through larger and larger veins and returns back to the heart, where the cycle restarts . . . .

The heart muscle (myocardium) contracts about 60 to 80 times a minute. During the contraction phase, or *systole,* blood is forced out of both ventricles. During the relaxation phase, or *diastole,* both ventricles fill up with blood coming from the atria. The system of valves keeps the blood moving in only one direction through the heart chambers. Actually, the heart is a double pump. As the ventricles contract (during systole), the mitral and tricuspid valves snap shut, preventing blood from flowing back into the atria. At the same time the aortic and pulmonic valves open and blood is forced under pressure into the aorta and pulmonary artery, respectively. Of course, the "two hearts" work at the same time, in coordinated fashion.

Blood pressure is the force of blood against the walls of the arteries, created by the heart as it pumps blood to all parts of the body. The walls of the arteries are elastic, so they stretch and then contract, to take the ups and downs of the blood pressure. When the blood pressure is taken, two pressures are recorded in numbers, for example 120/80. The "upper" number is the systolic pressure, generated when the heart contracts, and it measures how hard the left ventricle (the main pumping chamber) works to pump blood. The "lower" number is the diastolic pressure, produced when the heart relaxes between beats; it measures the resistance of the arteries to blood flow. The more difficult it is for the blood to flow through the arteries, the higher the pressure.

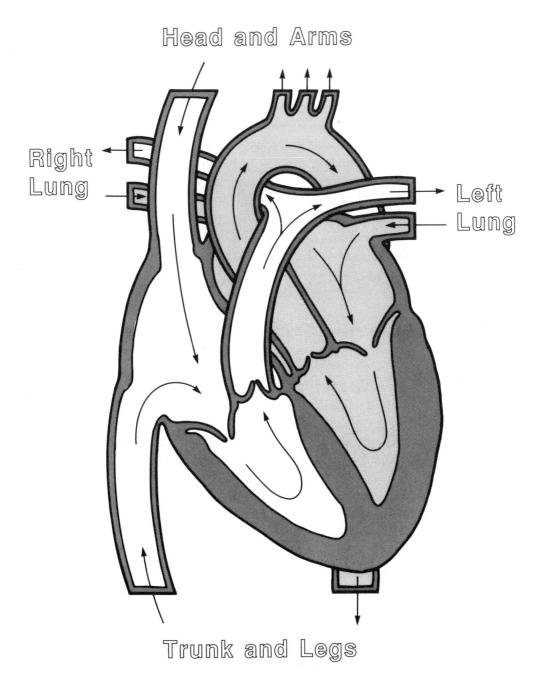

Figure 10. The circulatory system.

The pumping function of the heart is under the control of the *cardiac electrical system* that generates the electrical impulses necessary for the rhythmic contraction of the heart chambers . The sinus node, a small bundle of highly specialized cells, functions as a natural pacemaker, setting the pace for the heartbeat. (See figure 40, on page 192). The sinus node is located at the top of the right atrium, and from there the electrical signals radiate throughout the atria to the atrioventricular (AV) node, located at the junction of the atria and ventricles. From the AV node the electrical impulses are conducted through a conduction system made of specialized muscle fibers which then forks into the left and right bundle branches. Each bundle branch then divides into a network of smaller fibers which finally activate the corresponding ventricle. The electrical signals and currents within the heart regulate its rhythm, that is, the coordinated contraction of atria and ventricles.

The Coronary Arteries: Feeding the Heart Muscle

As we have seen, the heart is a hard-working pump. In order to accomplish its task, the heart muscle needs oxygen and nutrients. Although blood flows through its chambers, the heart cannot feed itself directly from inside the chambers. The blood vessels that supply the oxygen-rich blood to the heart muscle are the coronary arteries. They get their name from the Latin word "corona," which means crown, because they encircle the heart like a crown.

As blood leaves the left ventricle, it is forced into the body's main artery, the aorta, which arches over the top of the heart and then down through the chest and abdomen. At the very beginning of the aorta, near the top of the heart, arise the two coronary arteries, termed "left" and "right" coronary arteries. They travel on the surface of the heart, divide into smaller branches, and finally penetrate deep into the heart muscle, carrying oxygen-rich blood to the cells of the heart muscle. (See figure 11).

The initial segment of the left coronary artery, called the left main coronary artery, has the diameter of a drinking straw, and is less than an inch long. It is an extremely important blood vessel, since it conducts over two-thirds of the oxygen-rich blood feeding the heart muscle.

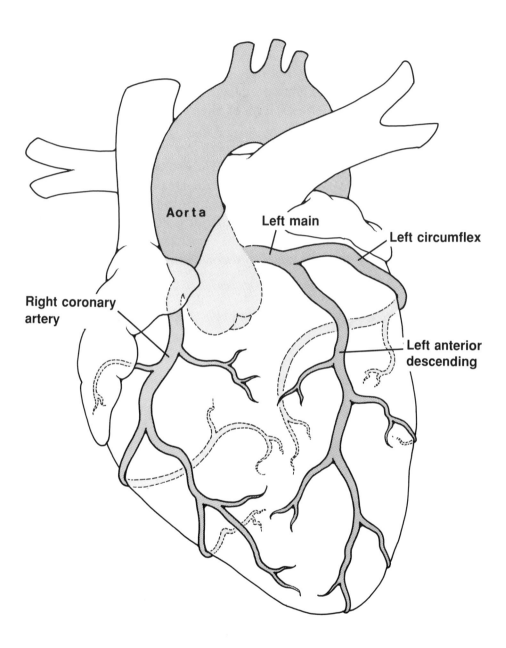

Figure 11. The coronary arteries.

The left main coronary artery branches into two slightly narrower arteries: the left anterior descending artery, which travels down the front of the heart, and the left circumflex artery, which circles around the left side, then to the back of the heart. The right coronary artery, which originates from the aorta, travels to the right side, then to the back of the heart. Doctors talk about the coronary arteries in term of three blood vessels: the two left arteries and the one right artery.

Most of the blood supplied by the coronary arteries goes to the left ventricle, the main pumping chamber. Each one of the three coronary arteries supplies oxygen-rich blood to a specific area of the left ventricular wall. The left anterior descending branch, for example, furnishes blood mainly to the front part of the ventricle (anterior wall); the left circumflex branch supplies blood to the side part of the ventricle (lateral wall); and the right coronary artery supplies blood to the underneath or back part of the ventricle (inferior wall).

As one can imagine, this marvelous pump, the heart, depends on the coronary arteries, since without the continuous supply of oxygen-rich blood it would not be able to perform its arduous task.

7 Symptoms of Heart Disease

Symptoms are warning signals sent by the body to inform us (and the doctor!) that a problem may exist within one of the body's systems. Symptoms must not be ignored, since this could place one's health and even life in jeopardy. Chest pain, for example, is often the first symptom of a heart attack. Ignoring this warning signal or waiting too long before seeking medical attention can prove to have serious consequences. The existence of a symptom, however, is not always indicative of a serious problem. Chest pain, for example, can result from a variety of non-cardiac conditions such as pleurisy, indigestion, arthritis, and anxiety, to mention just a few.

The four most common symptoms encountered in patients with heart disease are: chest pain, shortness of breath, palpitations, and fainting spell (syncope). These symptoms usually result from one or more of the following basic mechanisms (see figure 12): a) inadequate blood flow to the heart muscle; b) weakness of the heart pump; or c) disturbance of the cardiac rhythm.

Chest Pain

Chest pain is one of the most common symptoms in patients with heart disease. Chest pain, however, can be associated with many other non-cardiac conditions. A careful medical history is, without a doubt, the most important step toward defining the underlying problem. While taking the patient's history, the doctor will ask a series of questions concerning the characteristics of the discomfort, such as:

- What does it feel like? (pressure? sharp? burning? "gas?")
- Where is the pain located and where does it spread to? (chest? arms? back? neck?)
- How long does it usually last? (a few seconds? minutes? hours?)
- What brings it on? (exertion? emotional upset? a heavy meal?)
- Are there other associated symptoms? (nausea and vomiting? cold sweat? shortness of breath?)

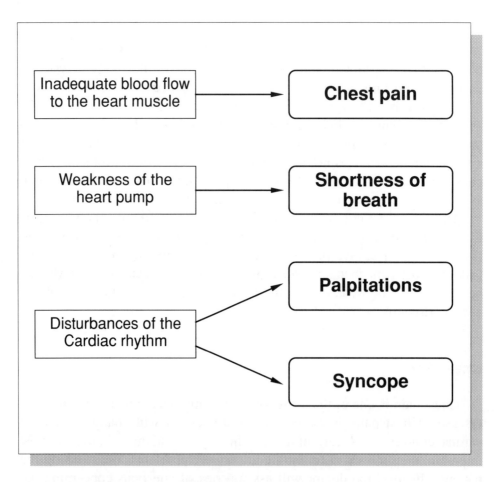

Figure 12. Common symptoms of heart disease and their underlying mechanisms.

The characteristics of the discomfort will often provide the doctor with clues about its possible underlying cause. Chest pain of angina, for example, is typically a squeezing or pressure type discomfort, located behind the sternum (breastbone); it usually occurs with exertion, lasts for a period of a few minutes, and is relieved by rest. The chest pain of a heart attack resembles that of angina in character and location, but is typically more severe, lasts longer, and does not subside with rest. Patients often break out in a cold sweat, feel weak and apprehensive, and may complain of shortness of breath, nausea and vomiting.

Chest pain is not necessarily due to heart disease. The pain can arise from other organs within the chest cavity (such as lungs, stomach, esophagus), or it can originate from the bony structures of the chest and spine. Great skill and good clinical judgement are often necessary in order to distinguish between medical emergencies (such as severe angina or heart attack) and other less urgent conditions. Here are some of the most common non-cardiac causes of chest pain:

• Disorders of the lungs: pleurisy, pneumonia, collapse of the lung, tumor of the lung.

• Disorders of the gastro-intestinal tract: hiatal hernia, esophagitis, ulcer of the stomach or duodenum, gallbladder disease.

• Disorders of the bones or muscles: arthritis of the spine, local chest wall pain, local inflammation of the rib joints, muscles, or ligaments.

• Emotional disorders: anxiety, tension, hyperventilation.

Shortness of Breath

Shortness of breath, or dyspnea, is an uncomfortable awareness of breathing. Patients may use a number of expressions to describe their discomfort: "difficulty breathing," "cannot get enough air," "air does not go all the way down," "tightness in the chest," or "choking sensation."

Shortness of breath is most commonly associated with diseases of the heart and lungs. Patients with chronic lung disease (chronic bronchitis and emphysema), for example, often have chronic symptoms of shortness of breath, recurrent cough, production of phlegm, and wheezing. These patients frequently have a long history of smoking cigarettes. Occasionally, shortness of breath can be seen with other conditions, such as marked obesity, anemia, and anxiety states.

When associated with heart disease, shortness of breath is usually the result of congestive heart failure, a condition in which the weakened heart is unable to pump enough blood to maintain adequate circulation, therefore leading to congestion of the lungs.

In most patients with congestive heart failure, shortness of breath occurs during exertion or activity (dyspnea on exertion), and is relieved by rest. In other patients, the discomfort occurs in the lying position (orthopnea), usually at night, and relief is obtained by sleeping with the head propped up on several pillows. Other patients may be suddenly awakened in the middle of the night with severe shortness of breath (paroxysmal nocturnal dyspnea), and they must sit on the edge of the bed or stand up for relief.

Palpitations

Palpitations is an unpleasant awareness of the beating of the heart. Normally, we are not aware of the rhythmic beating of the heart within the chest. However, when the cardiac rhythm becomes irregular, abnormally slow (bradycardia), or abnormally fast (tachycardia), we may become conscious of the heart beat.

The patient's description of the sensation may vary according to the type of rhythm disturbance. Premature contractions, for example, are often described as a "flopping sensation" in the chest or as "skipped beats." Tachycardia is usually described as a "fluttering sensation" or "racing heart," lasting for a period of minutes or sometimes hours.

The existence of palpitations does not necessarily mean the presence of a heart condition. Some patients complaining of recurrent palpitations, for example, may have a perfectly normal heart. The underlying problem in many of these patients is excessive anxiety and tension. Vice versa, some patients with significant documented arrhythmias may not complain of any symptoms. Obtaining an electrocardiogram (ECG) during the episode of palpitations, whenever feasible, is the best way to determine the nature of the rhythm disturbance.

Fainting Spell (Syncope)

Syncope is the medical term for a sudden loss of consciousness, or "fainting spell." When associated with heart disease, syncope results from a temporary reduction of blood flow and oxygen supply to the brain. This is most commonly caused by a variety of cardiac arrhythmias (such as an extremely slow or extremely fast heartbeat), or any condition that results in a sudden drop of the blood pressure.

Loss of consciousness is not always a symptom of heart disease. It can be seen with other non-cardiac disorders (such as epilepsy, stroke, hypoglycemia, anxiety attack, and hysterical fainting). The differentiation between these various conditions is often difficult, and a careful history obtained from the patient and accounts from witnesses are of great value.

At the onset of a typical syncopal attack the patient is in the sitting or standing position. He is usually warned of the impending faint by a sense of not feeling well, lightheadedness, and giddiness. His senses may become confused, spots may appear before the eyes, and vision may dim. Often there is a striking paleness or ashen gray color of the face, and quite often the face and body are bathed in cold perspiration. Because these symptoms precede loss of consciousness, the patient is often able to protect himself as he falls. If he can lie down promptly, the attack may be averted without complete loss of consciousness. The patient may remain in a state of unconsciousness for a few seconds to a few minutes. Once he is in a lying position, the gravitation no longer hinders the blood flow to the brain; the pulse becomes stronger, color begins to return to the face, and consciousness is regained.

When syncope is the result of a cardiac arrhythmia, it is due to either an extremely slow or extremely fast heartbeat, for example a heart rate below 40 per minute or over 200 per minute (normally, it is between 60 to 100 beats per minute). At these abnormal heart rates there is marked reduction of the amount of blood pumped by the heart, therefore leading to diminished blood flow to the brain, and eventually to loss of consciousness.

Near-syncope or "faintness" refers to a situation in which the person feels a sudden onset of dizziness and weakness, but does not lose consciousness. The episode is generally brief, lasting for only a few seconds, rarely over a minute. Simple dizziness is generally not the consequence of heart disease or cardiac arrhythmias; but when it is, it may signal a reduction in blood flow that is potentially serious.

Vasovagal syncope, or the "common faint," may be experienced by persons with a normal heart. It is often precipitated by an unpleasant stimulus such as fear, the sight of blood, or during a painful experience such as a venous puncture. It is most likely to occur in association with hunger, fatigue, or crowding, particularly in a hot room.

In *postural hypotension* there is a sudden fall of blood pressure when the patient sits up or stands up abruptly. This can result in severe dizziness or a brief loss of consciousness. Postural hypotension is commonly seen in patients recovering from a prolonged illness requiring bed rest, and in the elderly. It is also seen as a side effect from certain medications, especially those taken for the treatment of high blood pressure.

8 The Physician and the Diagnostic Process

Diagnosing heart disease involves a series of logical steps taken by the physician with the purpose of discovering the cause of the patient's problem. Years ago, in order to make an accurate diagnosis, the only data the physician had to rely on were his own observations and the patient's description of symptoms. Over the years, however, major scientific and technological advances began to emerge, and new techniques for the diagnosis of heart disease were developed, thus making the diagnostic process more complex.

Even with today's sophisticated technology, the patient's history remains the most valuable technique for determining whether or not his symptoms are caused by heart disease. The physical examination provides additional clues about the nature and possible causes of the patient's illness. Diagnostic tests are an extension of the patient history and physical examination; they allow the doctor to detect things that are not yet apparent and to confirm what is already suspected.

Proceeding in a series of logical steps, the physician uses his knowledge and his clinical judgment to analyze the different clinical findings, eventually reaching a conclusion — the diagnosis.

The Physician

American medicine is organized into a complex structure in which there are three broadly defined levels for the delivery of care. Primary care is a comprehensive and personal care that can be obtained by individuals on their own initiative, often without referral by another doctor. Secondary care is a higher level of care provided by a specialist or subspecialist. Access to this level generally requires a doctor's referral, although many patients now refer themselves. Tertiary care is highly specialized care, oriented toward complex problems and high-technology procedures. Care of this kind requires extended training on the part of physicians, sophisticated equipment for diagnosis and treatment, and specialized facilities.

Specialization is the almost inevitable response on the part of doctors to a field of knowledge that has become increasingly broad and complex. It provides the opportunity to master with competence a more limited body of material, and to feel confident in the application of that material to patient needs. Specialization has resulted in greatly improved health care, especially where serious illness is concerned. However, it has also resulted in fragmentation of care among specialists, and a decrease in long-term contact between individual doctors and patients.

The Primary Care Physician

The primary care physician is the one who oversees the patient's general health over a period of time, and who is familiar with the individual's complete medical history, living environment, and family situation. He is the one who refers the patient to the appropriate specialists, and then coordinates the recommendations and actions of the specialists involved in the case. Until a decade or two ago, the doctor selected as the primary-care physician was usually a general practitioner (GP). Such nonspecialists are now few, however, and their place has been gradually filled by internists and family practitioners.

The internist is a specialist in internal medicine, the branch of medicine that deals with the diagnosis and treatment of disorders of the internal organs (heart, lungs, kidneys, intestines, etc.). After having obtained the degree of Medical Doctor (MD), the internist's training includes an intensive program of graduate medical education (residency), generally in a hospital setting, for a period of at least three years. Internists are trained in the various subspecialty areas of internal medicine, as well as in the essential aspects of emergency medical care and critical care. The family practitioner has postgraduate training in internal medicine, as well as additional limited training in gynecology, pediatrics, and minor surgery.

The internist is primarily a diagnostician, a "medical detective," whose mark is thoroughness. During the initial visit, the internist obtains a comprehensive medical history, and then performs a thorough physical examination, searching for clues to a correct and complete diagnosis. When indicated, he may order one or more diagnostic tests, which are useful in further defining the nature of the problem. Most internists act as their patients' personal physician, conducting a continuing relationship with them. A large number of internists also act as consultants to other physicians, providing a diagnosis, an opinion, and recommendations for treatment in the various areas of internal medicine.

As recently as twenty years ago, the selection of the appropriate diagnostic tests in patients with heart disease was relatively easy, since the choices were limited to only two simple tests: the electrocardiogram (ECG) and the chest x-ray. With today's sophisticated technology and information explosion, however, the diagnostic process has become increasingly more complex, and no single doctor can now cope simultaneously with advances in all areas of internal medicine. As a result, today's internist will often need the advice and assistance of a heart specialist (cardiologist) to diagnose and manage the more complex forms of heart disease.

The Cardiologist

The cardiologist is a subspecialist in cardiology, the area of internal medicine that deals with the diagnosis and treatment of heart disease. The cardiologist's educational background includes an intensive residency program in internal medicine, taken over a period of three years or more (basically the same program a general internist goes through). In addition, the cardiologist trainee completes an intensive training program (cardiology fellowship), under the supervision of experienced cardiologists. The fellowship program, which usually takes two or three years, provides the physician with the necessary knowledge and skills needed to diagnose and manage complex types of heart disease.

The cardiologist is an expert diagnostician. He has the skills necessary to obtain a complete medical history and to perform a thorough physical examination, concentrating primarily on the cardiovascular system. In addition, he has the technical know-how to perform and interpret the various diagnostic tests available in the field of cardiology.

The practice of cardiology varies with the individual interests, training, and experience of each cardiologist. Most cardiologists practice as consultants, providing their opinion and recommendations to other physicians (mostly internists and family practitioners). Some cardiologists combine the practice of general internal medicine with the practice of consultative cardiology, thus providing primary care to their own patients as well as cardiology consultations for patients referred by other physicians.

Some cardiologists, finally, have restricted their practice to highly specialized care, oriented toward the interpretation of complex cardiac problems and performance of high-tech procedures (such as coronary balloon angioplasty). Obviously, care of this kind requires extensive training on the part of the cardiologist, sophisticated equipment, and specialized facilities.

Contrary to what many people think, the cardiologist is not a cardiac surgeon! He is primarily a diagnostician. Cardiac surgery is a highly sophisticated and complex kind of surgery, requiring a separate type of training and different skills. In the case of a patient with severe symptoms of angina (chest pain), for example, it is the cardiologist who establishes the diagnosis, by performing the appropriate diagnostic studies (such as exercise stress test and coronary angiography). If the patient is found to be a candidate for coronary bypass surgery, he will then be referred to a cardiac surgeon, who will review the findings and perform the operation.

The History and Physical

Even with today's technological advances, the patient's history remains the richest source of information in patients suspected of having heart disease. By taking a thorough history and listening closely to the patient's comments, the physician can help establish a bond with the patient and minimize the patient's apprehension and fear. It is largely upon such direct contact between patient and physician that confidence can be built. The physical examination follows the medical history, at the same session.

Patient History

When the physician is taking the history, the patient is first given the opportunity to relate his problem in his own words. The most common symptoms in patients with heart disease are chest pain, shortness of breath, and palpitations. After the patient has given an account of his present problem, the physician will ask specific questions regarding those symptoms, such as: frequency, intensity, aggravating factors, and response to treatment. He will then inquire about the presence or absence of other symptoms, and will ask questions about the patient's activities and physical limitations, if any.

Next, the physician will ask about major active medical problems, past medical history, history of surgery or injuries, medications being taken, and allergies to drugs. He will inquire about history of heart disease in the family, and the cause of death of parents and siblings. He will then perform a "review of systems," that is, a survey of specific symptoms (such as headaches, cough, vomiting, urinary problems, and joint pains, to mention just a few) relating to each of the major body systems. Finally, he will inquire about the person's overall lifestyle, such as type of work, pressure on the job, leisure activities, and personal habits (such as cigarette smoking, alcohol consumption, and dietary habits).

Physical Examination

The examination must be methodical and extend to all parts of the body, literally from head to toe, in a search for abnormalities that could yield important diagnostic information. In patients with heart disease, the physician will first perform a general examination, and will then direct his full attention to the cardiovascular system.

The pulse, resulting from the expansion and contraction of an artery, is usually checked at the wrist. It provides information about the heart rate (number of beats per minute) and rhythm (regular or irregular). The blood pressure, which represents the pressure of blood in the arteries, is then checked with blood pressure equipment.

The examination of the chest and lungs provides the physician with important information regarding the condition of the respiratory system. He will first percuss (thump) with his fingers over the back looking for areas of dullness, which can indicate an abnormal collection of fluid between the lungs and the chest wall. He will then auscultate (listen to) the patient's breath sounds with his stethoscope. In patients with congestive heart failure the lungs become congested, and crackling sounds (called rales) can be heard over the lower portion of the chest.

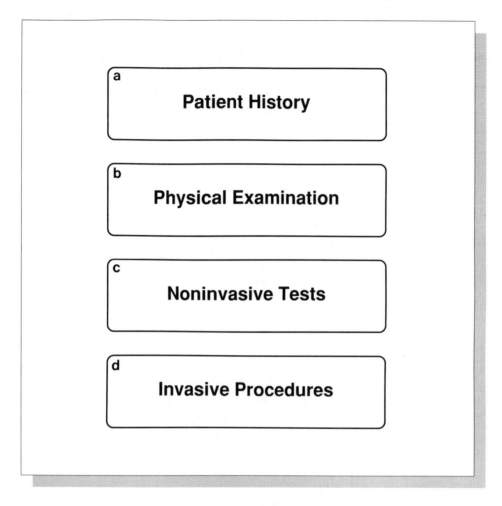

Figure 13. The basic steps of the diagnostic process.

The next step, the most important in patients with heart disease, is the examination of the heart itself. Using his stethoscope, the physician will perform a careful cardiac auscultation, listening over several areas of the chest, in order to obtain maximum information. The normal heart sounds (called "first" and "second" heart sounds) have often been described as "lub, dub. . . lub, dub." They result from the sudden closure of the heart valves during the different phases of the cardiac contraction.

Abnormal heart sounds (such as "gallop," "click," and "snap") usually represent either weakness of the heart pump or a defect of the heart valves. Heart murmurs result from turbulence in the blood stream, and often represent a malformed or defective valve. It should be emphasized that abnormal heart sounds or heart murmurs can sometimes be heard in healthy persons. The reverse is also true, whereby some patients with severe heart disease may have normal heart sounds on auscultation.

The physician then examines the abdomen, especially the liver, which may become congested and enlarged in cases of severe heart failure. He will then inspect the lower extremities for the presence of edema (swelling), which in some patients may be a manifestation of congestive heart failure. The careful and systematic examination of the peripheral arterial pulses in the extremities and the neck is very important in the patient with heart disease. A weak or absent pulse in the leg, for example, may represent narrowing or blockage of the artery supplying blood to that leg.

Diagnostic Tests and Procedures

Based on the data obtained during the medical history and physical examination, the physician will determine whether further diagnostic studies are needed in order to make an accurate diagnosis.

Tests used for the diagnosis of heart disease can be classified into two general categories: noninvasive tests, which do not involve the insertion of devices into the patient's body; and invasive procedures, which do require the insertion of catheters and other devices into the patient's body. Although noninvasive tests are safer, invasive procedures are usually far more detailed and accurate in providing diagnostic information.

The proper combination of tests will generally provide the physician with enough information to make a meaningful diagnosis. Choosing the most appropriate tests for the individual patient, however, is not always easy. The physician must have sufficient knowledge in the field of medicine, and most importantly, he must possess good clinical judgment, that is, the ability to clearly formulate a clinical problem and to proceed in an orderly manner to its solution.

⑨ Noninvasive Diagnostic Tests

Noninvasive tests do not involve the insertion of devices into the patient's body. They are therefore safer than invasive procedures. Tests commonly used for the diagnosis of heart disease include: electrocardiogram (ECG), chest x-ray, echocardiogram, ambulatory ECG monitoring (Holter), exercise stress test (treadmill), and nuclear scanning.

Most patients with heart-related symptoms will require at least two basic tests: an ECG and a chest x-ray. When the diagnosis cannot be established with these basic tests, additional tests will be performed.

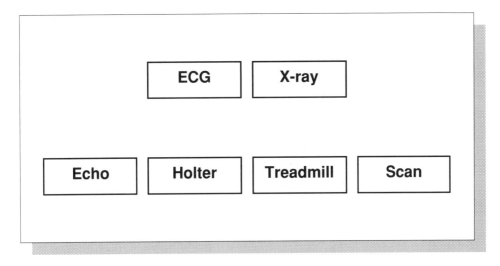

Figure 14. Noninvasive tests used in the diagnosis of heart disease.

Electrocardiogram (ECG or EKG)

The electrocardiogram is a graphic recording of the electrical activity produced in association with the heartbeat. The electrical impulses generated and conducted within the heart result in weak electrical currents that spread through the entire body. These electrical impulses are amplified and recorded by the ECG apparatus. The test allows the physician to identify any changes in the pattern of the electrical deflections that may indicate the presence of heart disease which has occurred in the past or is occurring in the present.

The test itself involves the placement of several electrodes (small metal discs) on the patient's chest, arms, and legs. These electrodes are connected by wires to the ECG machine. The electrical impulses cause a special needle to move over a strip of moving paper and record the heartbeat as a wavy line.

The ECG tracing is a combination of deflections, above and below the baseline, representing the electrical events within the heart. (See figure 15). The small initial wave of the ECG, called the P wave, represents the electrical activation of the atria (the upper heart chambers). Next comes the QRS complex, the tallest deflection on the ECG, representing the activation of the ventricles. Finally, the T wave represents the recovery period of the ventricles, when they recharge their spent electrical forces.

The ECG test is useful in diagnosing cardiac arrhythmias (disturbances of the cardiac rhythm). Normally, the heart rate is between 60 to 100 beats per minute and the rhythm is regular. During a cardiac arrhythmia, the heart rate may be too slow (bradycardia) or too fast (tachycardia), or the rhythm may be irregular. By carefully examining the tracing, the physician can diagnose the majority of cardiac arrhythmias (see Chapter 17). All too often, however, arrhythmias are transient and may not occur during the brief period of recording. A person complaining of only occasional palpitations, for example, may have a perfectly normal tracing during the actual recording. If the presence of an arrhythmia is strongly suspected, the doctor may order an ambulatory ECG monitoring (see page 92).

The ECG is also used for the diagnosis of chamber enlargement, often present in patients with long-standing or severe heart disease. Enlargement of the left atrium, for example, will result in widening of the P wave.

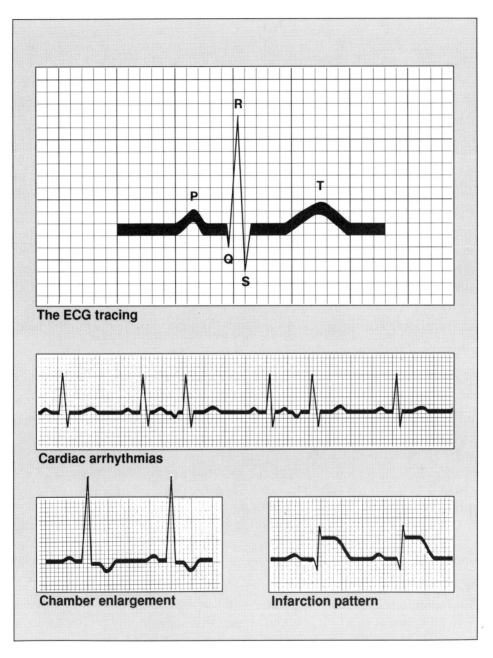

The ECG tracing

Cardiac arrhythmias

Chamber enlargement

Infarction pattern

Figure 15. The ECG tracing is a combination of deflections that represent the electrical events within the heart. It is most useful for diagnosing cardiac arrhythmias, chamber enlargement, and myocardial infarction.

Enlargement of the left ventricle or thickening (hypertrophy) of the ventricular wall, on the other hand, will result in increased size of the QRS complex. Although useful in detecting the presence of chamber enlargement or hypertrophy, the ECG is not very helpful in assessing the severity of the problem. When a more accurate measurement of chamber dimensions and wall thickness is required, the doctor may order additional tests, such as an echocardiogram (see page 89).

The ECG is of particular value in the diagnosis of acute myocardial infarction ("fresh" heart attack). Serial tracings obtained over a course of several days will usually show a series of typical changes. These changes represent abnormalities of the electrical currents within the heart, resulting from injury and damage to the heart muscle. In the initial hours after a heart attack, there is typically an elevation of the ST segment (the segment between the QRS complex and the T wave), representing injury to the heart muscle. Several hours or days later, there is appearance of abnormal Q waves, representing the infarction (permanent tissue damage). Since they represent dead scar tissue, these abnormal Q waves will persist indefinitely on future tracings.

The ECG is generally not helpful in the diagnosis of angina (a condition resulting from inadequate blood supply to the heart muscle), since the test is normal or nearly normal in over half of these patients. In fact, patients suffering from typical angina symptoms during exertion can have a normal ECG at rest. For this reason, whenever angina is suspected, the doctor may order an exercise stress test (see page 94).

The ECG is an easily conducted test that can be done in the doctor's office or in a hospital bed. The test itself takes less than fifteen minutes and it is not associated with any risk or discomfort.

The ECG is only a laboratory test, and as such it must always be interpreted in the light of other clinical findings. A normal ECG does not exclude the possibility of severe heart disease! For example, a patient with severe narrowing of the coronary arteries may have a perfectly normal ECG. The reverse is also true: a person with an abnormal ECG may have a perfectly normal heart. It is a known fact that some highly trained athletes (especially long-distance runners) may have significant abnormalities on their ECG, due to the enlargement of their heart from the endurance training (so-called "athlete's heart").

Chest X-ray

X-rays are a form of radiant energy that can pass "through" objects. Like light rays, they cause silver to precipitate (deposit) on photographic film, and therefore blacken the film. X-rays travel freely through air but are absorbed by certain objects, such as metal and bone. Air-filled objects allow most of the rays to reach the film and will therefore appear black. Dense objects, on the other hand, absorb most of the x-rays, and will appear white. The form and shape of the x-ray "shadows" allows one to make reasonable and useful deductions regarding the objects in question.

The chest x-ray shows dense structures (such as spine and ribs) in white, and air-filled tissues (such as lungs) in black. (See figure 16). The heart and major blood vessels have an intermediate x-ray density, resulting in a light-grey appearance. The contours of the "cardiac silhouette" (heart shadow) are clearly outlined because they contrast with the adjacent air-containing lungs, which are black. Only those chambers and blood vessels that form a border on any particular view can be seen and evaluated. Structures within the heart (such as chambers, walls, and valves) cannot be seen.

A chest x-ray is usually included in the initial evaluation of most patients suspected of having heart disease. The appearance of the heart and lungs on a chest x-ray film often provides clues regarding the presence or absence of cardiac abnormalities. In patients with known heart disease, the chest x-ray is helpful in assessing the severity of the condition, and in documenting the progression of the disease or its response to treatment.

The chambers of the heart and the large blood vessels (aorta and pulmonary artery) always occupy the same relative position within the cardiac silhouette. The enlargement of any of these structures will affect the contours of the heart in a fairly characteristic manner, thus helping the doctor to identify the structure involved. Enlargement of the left ventricle (the main pumping chamber), for example, will result in widening of the lower part of the cardiac silhouette. Dilatation (enlargement) of the aorta (the body's main artery), on the other hand, will result in widening of the top part of the silhouette.

The chest x-ray is not always helpful. Different cardiac disorders can result in similar findings on the x-ray film. When fluid is present around the heart (pericardial effusion), for example, the widening of the heart shadow

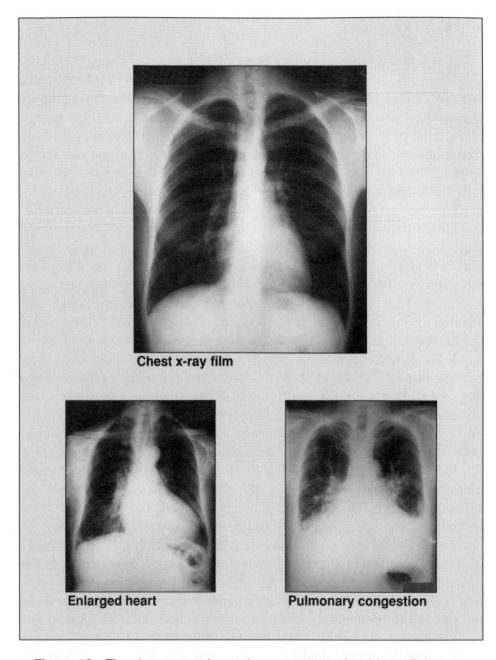

Chest x-ray film

Enlarged heart

Pulmonary congestion

Figure 16. The chest x-ray shows dense structures in white or light grey, and air-filled structures (lungs) in black. It is most useful for estimating the heart size and for detecting pulmonary congestion.

will be somewhat similar to that seen with enlargement of the left ventricle. In fact, it may be difficult or even impossible to differentiate the two conditions. Other times, a significant deformity of a cardiac structure will cause minimal change on the x-ray. Patients with abnormal thickening (hypertrophy) of the heart muscle, for example, often appear to have a normal size heart on the chest x-ray. As the heart muscle thickens, it tends to encroach on the chamber cavity, and therefore may not cause a significant change in the shape of the cardiac silhouette.

After having carefully examined the shape of the heart and its size, the doctor will inspect the "lung fields," which contain the lung tissue and the pulmonary blood vessels (arteries, veins, and capillaries). In patients with congestive heart failure, the lungs become congested and fill up with fluid. Since the x-ray density of fluid is denser than that of the lung tissue itself, there will be the appearance of small white patchy areas within the lung fields (pulmonary congestion).

The chest x-ray is a simple and relatively non-expensive test, and it can often be done in the doctor's office. The amount of radiation during the brief exposure is minimal and of no consequence (except in pregnant women, in whom x-rays should be avoided, if possible).

The major limitation of the chest x-ray is its inability to visualize the structures inside the heart, such as the chamber cavities, the ventricular walls, and the heart valves. When there is a need to better define these cardiac structures, the doctor may order a more sophisticated technique, such as the echocardiogram (see below).

Echocardiogram

The echocardiogram is a technique that utilizes ultrasound waves to examine the heart structures. It is an extremely useful test for the diagnosis of various forms of heart disease. The technique is somewhat similar to that of sonar, which is used by ships to determine the depth and location of underwater objects. A short burst of ultrasound is beamed through the chest wall. When it strikes a boundary line between two tissues with different acoustic properties, the ultrasound wave is reflected back toward the surface, where it can be recorded.

During the test, a small cylindrical device (transducer) is placed on the patient's chest wall, just left of the sternum (breastbone). The transducer functions both as a transmitter of ultrasound waves and as a receiver, "reading" the time elapsed between transmission and reception of the reflected sound waves. A computer converts these "echoes" into an image of the heart's interior, thus showing the motion of the heart valves and the contraction of the cardiac chambers. By manipulating the transducer in various directions, a variety of structures can be visualized, and a display of their motion can then be recorded. (See figure 17).

The complete study is actually a combination of two different but complementary techniques. In the original technique, termed *M-mode echocardiography,* the tracing is displayed on a strip of paper. Ultrasound waves reflected from the heart are displayed on a time chart recording, with depth on the vertical axis and time on the horizontal axis. This technique has proved extremely valuable for measuring the size of the cardiac chambers and thickness of the walls, and for visualizing the fast motion of the heart valves. The major limitation of the M-mode method is that it does not permit evaluation of the actual shape of the heart structures.

A more advanced technique, called *two-dimensional echocardiography* (or simply "two-D echo"), has become popular because it provides some of the information not available with the M-mode technique. This sophisti-cated technique can show the actual shape of the different cardiac structures as well as their actual motion. In a way, the two-D images represent individual "slices" of the heart in motion. Such recordings can be displayed on a small television screen and stored on videotapes.

A newer technique, called *Doppler echocardiography,* is now available for evaluating the velocity (speed) of blood within the heart chambers. The Doppler technique is quite useful in assessing the abnormal turbulent flow patterns resulting from defective (narrowed or leaky) valves.

The echocardiogram can be performed in the doctor's office, or at the hospital. It is a safe technique, which takes about 30 minutes to complete, and has no discomfort or risk to the patient. It is a relatively expensive test, but it provides invaluable information that often cannot be obtained by any other technique. The major limitation of echocardiography is that a good quality image is often difficult to obtain in patients who are obese, and in those suffering from chronic lung disease (emphysema).

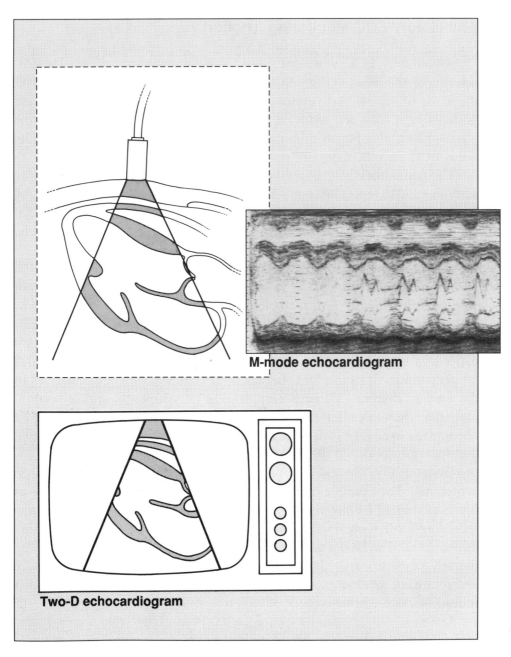

M-mode echocardiogram

Two-D echocardiogram

Figure 17. The echocardiogram is a technique that utilizes ultrasound waves to examine the heart structures. The complete study is actually a combination of two different but complementary techniques.

Ambulatory ECG Monitoring (Holter)

Ambulatory ECG monitoring is a 24-hour recording of the electrical activity of the heart. The test is especially useful in the detection and diagnosis of cardiac arrhythmias. The Holter monitor itself is a light and portable tape recorder, worn on a strap over the shoulder or around the waist. Electrodes (small discs) are placed on the patient's chest, and the wires from the electrodes are plugged into the recorder.

The patient being monitored is instructed to engage in his usual daily activities and to report in a diary any symptoms he may develop. Following the recording, the tape is played back at fast speed and scanned by a special computer for abnormalities and irregularities. Cardiac arrhythmias can be detected this way, and the time of their occurrence can be correlated with the patient's reported activities and symptoms. (See figure 18).

The main use for Holter monitoring is the detection of intermittent cardiac arrhythmias. For example, patients may complain of symptoms suggestive of an arrhythmia, such as palpitations, dizziness or faintness. Since these symptoms are often intermittent, an ECG done at the doctor's office may be perfectly normal. The Holter monitor, recorded over a much longer period will have a far better chance of detecting the abnormalities of the cardiac rhythm. Patients complaining of symptoms during specific activities (such as exercise, emotional stress, or sexual intercourse) will be encouraged to engage in those activities during the recording period, so that the rhythm response to the natural stress can be evaluated.

Occasionally, the test may be indicated in patients who may have no symptoms. For example, patients recovering from a heart attack are at an increased risk of having significant cardiac arrhythmias. For this reason, a recording is often obtained in such patients, soon after their discharge from the hospital. The Holter technique is also useful in patients placed on drug therapy for cardiac arrhythmias. The number of cardiac irregularities before and following treatment can be compared, thus providing the doctor with a tool to assess the effectiveness of different antiarrhythmic drugs.

More recently, the Holter technique has been used to diagnose myocardial ischemia (inadequate blood supply to the heart muscle) in patients suspected of having coronary heart disease. Most patients with coronary artery disease will develop abnormal ECG changes during periods of chest

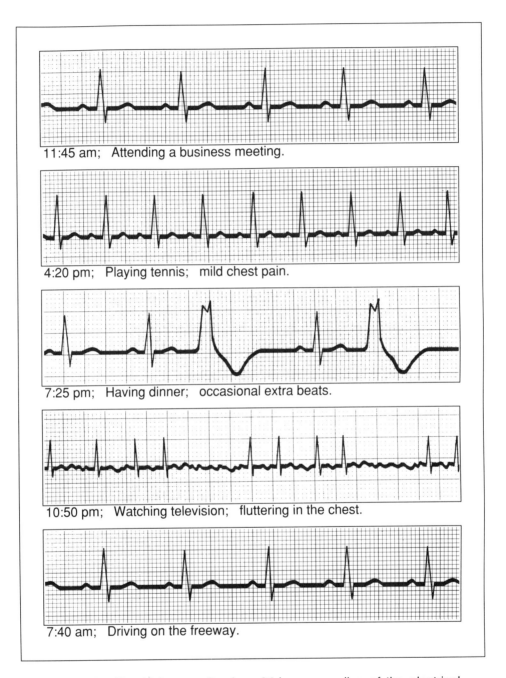

11:45 am; Attending a business meeting.

4:20 pm; Playing tennis; mild chest pain.

7:25 pm; Having dinner; occasional extra beats.

10:50 pm; Watching television; fluttering in the chest.

7:40 am; Driving on the freeway.

Figure 18. The Holter monitor is a 24-hour recording of the electrical activity of the heart. The occurrence of arrhythmias is then correlated with the patient's reported activities and symptoms.

pain (angina). In some patients, however, the ECG shows intermittent changes during the recording but without accompanying chest pain. This finding, termed "silent ischemia," may prove helpful for the detection of patients with severe coronary heart disease who, for some reason, do not develop any warning symptoms of angina.

The Holter technique is perfectly safe and is associated with only minimal inconvenience to the patient. It is a relatively expensive test (compared to an ECG) since it requires sophisticated computerized equipment for the rapid scanning of the recording. The main use of the Holter monitor is in the diagnosis of cardiac arrhythmias. Although it is used occasionally in the diagnosis of coronary heart disease, it is not as reliable for this purpose as the exercise stress test.

Exercise Stress Test (Treadmill)

The exercise stress test is a means of applying stress to the heart under controlled conditions. The way in which the heart tolerates the extra workload provides important information about its functional status. Some patients with significant coronary heart disease, for example, may not have any symptoms or ECG abnormalities in the resting state, but will develop them during exercise. The exercise stress test is therefore helpful in uncovering potential problems that may not be detected otherwise.

Prior to the stress test, the patient is informed of the indications, the potential benefits, as well as the possible risks. He is then asked to sign a written consent form. Several electrodes are placed on the patient's chest, to allow recording of the ECG during the exercise and to monitor the heart rate. The diagnostic testing must be supervised by a trained physician, usually an internist or cardiologist.

The patient is asked to walk on a motor-driven treadmill (or in some cases to ride a stationary bicycle) for a period of up to 15 minutes. The speed and the incline of the treadmill are increased every 3 minutes, according to a preset program (protocol). The patient is instructed to report any symptoms, such as chest pain, shortness of breath, fatigue, or dizziness. The blood pressure is checked every few minutes, and the ECG is carefully observed for abnormalities, such as ischemia (which result from inadequate blood supply to the heart muscle) or cardiac arrhythmias.

The exercise period is divided into several stages, each lasting for three minutes. The treadmill starts slowly, and then the speed and the grade (incline) gradually increase at each new stage. In the most frequently used program (called the Bruce protocol), the initial speed is 1.7 miles per hour and the initial grade is 10 degrees. During the fourth stage of the Bruce protocol (between the ninth and twelfth minutes) the speed is 4.2 miles and the grade is up to 16 degrees. The average healthy middle-age person is usually able to complete three stages (9 minutes) on this protocol.

The maximum heart rate that a patient can achieve during the treadmill test is "predicted" prior to the test itself. Generally, the maximum heart rate one can attain during strenuous exercise gradually decreases with age, meaning it is highest in children and lowest in the elderly. The maximum predicted heart rate can be approximated by subtracting the person's age from the number 220. As a safety measure, the test is usually terminated when the heart rate reaches about 90 percent of the maximum heart rate. For example, for a 50-year-old person, the predicted maximum heart rate is 220 minus 50, or 170 beats per minute. The "target" heart rate to be achieved during the test will be 170 times 90%, or 153 beats per minute.

The decision regarding the termination of the procedure is made by the physician supervising the test. He may stop the treadmill when the target heart rate has been achieved, or when the patient is unable to continue because of fatigue, shortness of breath, or chest pain. Other times, the test will be stopped because of abnormal changes on the ECG, or because of significant cardiac arrhythmias.

Exercise stress testing is a very helpful aid in the diagnosis of angina and evaluation of chest pain in adults. Angina results from inadequate blood supply to the heart muscle (ischemia), caused by the narrowing of one or more coronary arteries. During exercise, the heart performs extra work and thus temporarily needs more oxygen. Since the coronary blood flow is already limited by the narrowing, the oxygen supply becomes inadequate and this results in ischemia.

An ECG taken during a period of ischemia will usually (but not always) display abnormal changes in the form of ST segment depression, that is, lowering of the segment between the QRS complex and the T wave. (See figure 19). If the ECG changes during exercise suggest ischemia, especially if they are associated with symptoms of chest pain, the test is considered "positive." Although one may think that "positive" means a favorable

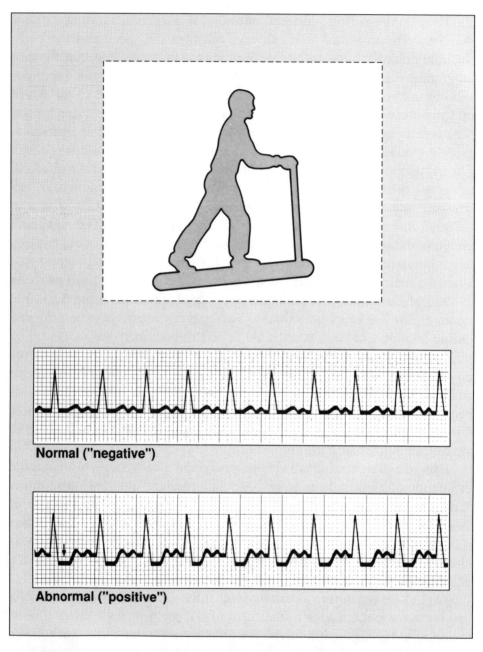

Normal ("negative")

Abnormal ("positive")

Figure 19. The treadmill stress test is particularly useful in the diagnosis of angina. An ECG taken during a period of ischemia will usually display abnormal changes in the form of ST segment depression.

result, in this case it means that coronary heart disease may be present. Actually, the desired result from a stress test is a "negative" one!

The stress test is a very useful diagnostic tool for the assessment of chest pain, especially when the clinical presentation is not entirely typical of angina. Even when the diagnosis appears certain from the patient's description of symptoms, the test is frequently used in order to assess the severity of the problem and determine the approach to treatment.

A treadmill test is also helpful in guiding rehabilitation of patients following a heart attack or coronary bypass surgery. Many physicians, for example, routinely perform a low level stress test in patients recovering from a heart attack, often prior to their discharge from the hospital. The results of the test help the physician to select the proper level of exercise that can be performed safely at home. In addition, the test is useful in identifying those patients who may be at a higher risk of having problems during the early stages of their recovery.

A treadmill is often recommended as a precautionary measure in sedentary persons over the age of 40 who contemplate a strenuous physical fitness program. Some doctors use it as a screening test in non-symptomatic patients who have one or more significant risk factors for coronary heart disease (such as heavy cigarette smoking, high blood pressure, high cholesterol level, or a family history of heart disease).

The stress test can be performed in the physician's office, or at the hospital. The test is relatively expensive (compared to a resting ECG), since it requires the use of a motorized treadmill and sophisticated ECG equipment. The exercise stress test has an excellent safety record. There is, however, a small amount of risk. Possible rare complications include cardiac arrhythmias, prolonged chest pain, and heart attack.

The major limitation of the exercise stress test is that it is not totally reliable, and it can sometimes give false results. A patient with documented coronary heart disease (by angiogram), for example, may have a negative (normal) treadmill; this is termed a "false negative" test. The other way around, a person with perfectly normal coronary arteries may have a positive (abnormal) treadmill; it is then termed a "false positive" test. When properly performed, the treadmill stress test has an accuracy of about 80 percent. The accuracy of the stress test can be improved by performing a simultaneous cardiac scan (see below).

Cardiac Nuclear Scanning

A cardiac scan is a noninvasive technique, in which a radioactive substance is injected into the bloodstream for the purpose of assessing the function of the heart. The gamma rays originating from the radioactive substance are detected by a gamma camera, and the information is processed with a sophisticated computer. The resulting image is a map of the distribution of radioactivity within the heart.

The cardiac scanning techniques are especially useful in the diagnosis of coronary heart disease and angina. The small amount of radioactive compound used for these tests is active for only a few hours, and can safely circulate in the bloodstream without causing any adverse reactions. The only potential risk may result from the exercise stress test used in combination with the scan. These techniques are available only in large hospitals and clinics, and are quite expensive, since they require costly equipment and sophisticated computers.

Two basic imaging techniques, each employing a different radioactive agent, are currently available for the diagnosis of heart disease and angina. Each of these two techniques provides a somewhat different type of information about the heart function.

a) Thallium Scan

This technique, also called myocardial imaging, is useful in the diagnosis of coronary heart disease and angina. It is usually performed in combination with a standard treadmill stress test. Thallium-201 is a radioactive substance taken up by the heart muscle in proportion to the coronary blood flow. During the test, the patient exercises on the treadmill for several minutes. A small amount of the substance is then injected into a vein while the patient is still on the treadmill. The radioactive thallium is carried in the bloodstream and diffuses into the heart muscle, mostly into areas well supplied with blood, as opposed to areas with ischemia (inadequate blood supply).

Following the exercise, the patient lies down on a test table and the imaging process begins. Areas of the heart muscle not getting enough blood will pick up little or no radioactivity. The pictures obtained reflect the blood

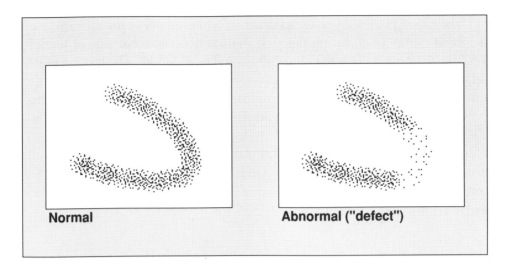

Normal

Abnormal ("defect")

Figure 20. The thallium scan is especially useful in the diagnosis of angina. The pictures obtained reflect the blood supply pattern to the heart muscle, showing "defects" in areas of ischemia.

supply pattern within the heart muscle, showing "cold spots" (or "defects") in areas of inadequate blood flow. (See figure 20).

The imaging is repeated a few hours later, to help differentiate between areas of transient ischemia (the defect is "reversible") and areas of permanent scarring from an old infarction (the defect is "irreversible").

b) Blood Pool Scan

This test, also called radioisotope ventriculogram, is useful in the noninvasive evaluation of the pumping function of the heart, and in the diagnosis of coronary heart disease. In this technique, red blood cells are tagged (labeled) with technetium (a radioactive substance) and then reinjected into the bloodstream through a vein in the arm. The radioactive substance, which is attached to the red blood cells, stays inside the circulation ("blood pool") and travels through the heart chambers. Imaging is performed with a gamma camera, and the data are processed with a sophisticated computer, providing a picture of the left ventricle during its actual contraction and relaxation.

The blood pool scan gives accurate information about the efficiency of the heart pump, by allowing the physician to observe the image of the left ventricle (the main pumping chamber) as it pumps blood. The motion of the different portions of the ventricular wall can be visualized (this part of the test is called "wall motion study"). If damage to the heart muscle has occurred, the wall will not contract normally, and this will show on the scan. The test is usually combined with an exercise stress test (on a stationary bicycle), thus providing information about the ventricular function during exercise. In patients with coronary heart disease, the test may be normal at rest, but will show abnormal function of the ventricle during exercise, when the heart muscle is ischemic ("starving" for oxygen).

· · · · · · ·

How Much Does It Cost?

The cost of diagnostic tests is highly variable, and depends on several factors, including where it's performed (office vs. hospital) and geographic location. The following list reflects the cost of commonly used diagnostic cardiac tests, in Southern California, during 1987. This list, which provides only general representative figures, is intended solely as a general reference.

Electrocardiogram	$50
Chest x-ray	$50
Holter monitor (24 hours)	$300
Exercise stress test	$300
Echocardiogram	$400
Thallium scan (including the treadmill)	$1,200
Cardiac catheterization & coronary angiography (including hospital charges & physician fees)	$5,000

10 Invasive Cardiac Procedures

Cardiac catheterization and coronary angiography are "invasive" procedures that involve the insertion of catheters and other devices into the patient's body. These procedures allow the physician to measure the actual pressures within the heart and blood vessels, and to visualize the coronary arteries (the arteries feeding the heart muscle) and the heart chambers.

In general, invasive procedures provide more accurate and detailed diagnostic information than noninvasive tests. Despite their accuracy, however, they cannot be recommended to every patient suspected of having heart disease. First of all, they are expensive and usually require a brief hospitalization. In addition, they entail a certain degree of risk.

During these procedures, a thin and flexible plastic tube, called a catheter, is inserted into a peripheral vein or artery (in the groin or arm) and then directed through larger blood vessels toward the central circulation and the heart. The progression of the catheter inside the body can be followed with the aid of special x-ray equipment.

Cardiac catheterization and coronary angiography each provide a somewhat different kind of diagnostic information. These techniques are complementary, however, and they are often combined into one procedure. Cardiac catheterization is used primarily to measure the pressures within the heart chambers and to assess the pumping function of the heart. During coronary angiography, a special radiographic dye (contrast) that can be seen with x-rays is injected through the catheter directly into the coronary arteries, providing a detailed picture of the coronary arteries. Contrast can also be injected into the ventricle (pumping chamber), thus giving additional information about the pumping function of the heart.

Before the Procedure

The patient is generally admitted to the hospital on the day prior to the procedure (in some cases, the patient arrives in the morning, on the day of the procedure). After admission formalities have been completed, the patient is escorted to his room in the cardiology ward. There, a unit nurse will familiarize him with the hospital routine, and will take his vital signs (pulse, blood pressure, and temperature). Several routine laboratory tests are performed soon after admission, including an ECG, a chest x-ray, and blood tests.

The physician who will perform the procedure (usually a cardiologist) reviews the medical history and examines the patient. He will then explain to the patient about the procedure, its purpose, the potential benefits, as well as the possible risks. The patient will then be asked to sign a consent form, which is essentially a legal document that gives permission to the doctor to perform the procedure. "Informed consent" means that the patient is fully aware of the potential benefits, possible risks, and the alternatives before he agrees to the procedure.

If the procedure is scheduled for the next morning, no food or drink is allowed after midnight. If it is scheduled for the next afternoon, a light breakfast may be permitted. The area of the groin (the fold where the thigh joins the trunk) is then cleansed and shaved, in order to facilitate the insertion of the catheters during the procedure and avoid infection. An intravenous (IV) line is inserted into a vein in the arm, and kept open by a slow infusion of glucose solution. This line will allow administration of drugs directly into the vein during the procedure, if needed. Mild sedation (either orally or by injection) is generally given within an hour before the patient leaves the room en route to the cardiac catheterization laboratory; this is done to alleviate apprehension and reduce anxiety.

During the Procedure

Cardiac catheterization and coronary angiography are performed in a specially equipped x-ray room, called a cardiac catheterization laboratory, or simply "cath lab." The patient is transported from his hospital room to the cath lab on a movable bed. He is then gently transferred to an x-ray table

What to Ask the Doctor Before a Test

The use of new sophisticated techniques and procedures has enhanced our ability to detect and diagnose various types of heart disease. These techniques, however, are costly and may entail a certain degree of discomfort and risk. It is the doctor's role to inform the patient about the indications for the test and the potential risk involved. It is the patient's responsibility, however, to be sure he really understands the doctor's recommendations, and to ask questions about anything that may not be clear. Here are some basic questions a patient should ask the doctor before undergoing a test:

• *Why is the test being ordered?* A diagnostic test can be ordered for several different reasons: to confirm a suspected diagnosis; to assess the severity of the problem; to rule out the presence of a potentially serious condition; to screen for a disease that has no symptoms; or sometimes to reassure the patient that a certain condition is not present.

• *Is there any pain or discomfort?* Most cardiac tests are painless or cause only brief discomfort, such as a needle puncture or the need to lie still for the length of the test. Invasive cardiac procedures are generally not painful, although some patients may report some discomfort during the manipulation of the catheters. Most of the discomfort is due to the need to lie still for a long period of time.

• *What is the risk involved?* Most noninvasive tests have no risk at all. The exercise stress test has an excellent safety record, but may be associated with a small amount of risk. Cardiac catheterization and coronary angiography are invasive procedures requiring insertion of a catheter that actually enters the body, and are therefore associated with a definite (although relatively small) risk.

• *What is the risk of not having the test?* The consequences of an undiagnosed illness may be much worse than the potential risk from the procedure. Not properly diagnosing the cause of chest pain can be of serious consequence. A patient refusing a coronary angiogram just because it is "too risky," for example, may lead to a potentially far more serious problem, such as a heart attack.

that has a large x-ray camera above it and a television screen close by. The equipment in the cath lab also includes monitors and various instruments and devices. There are usually four or five persons in the cath lab for the duration of the procedure: the cardiologist, an assistant, a nurse, and one or two technicians. In order to prevent contamination of the catheterization "field," the patient is draped with sterile sheets, and the staff wear sterile gowns and gloves.

The catheterization procedure involves the insertion of one or more catheters into a vein or artery in the groin area. (See figure 21). The area of insertion is cleansed thoroughly, and a local anesthetic is injected into the skin with a small needle, to numb the area. This may cause a mild stinging sensation (like a "mosquito bite"). A tiny incision is made in the skin, and a large needle is used to puncture the vein or artery. A soft and flexible metallic guide wire is inserted into the blood vessel, and the catheter is then slipped over the guide wire. Once the catheter is inside the blood vessel, the cardiologist slowly advances it toward the heart while watching its progress on the television screen.

(In some instances, the catheter(s) may be inserted in the arm, at the crease of the elbow. When using the arm approach, an incision (cut-down) about an inch wide is made to expose the blood vessels, and the catheter is inserted directly into the vein or artery, then advanced toward the heart).

Right heart catheterization is the part of the procedure that explores the "right side" of the heart. A special catheter with a small air-filled balloon at its tip is inserted into a *vein* and then advanced inside the circulation. The light-weight catheter tip "floats" with the blood flow, following the normal course taken by the blood when returning to the heart. As it is pushed, the catheter first advances toward the central veins, then toward the right atrium and right ventricle. If pushed further, the tip of the catheter will go across the pulmonic valve, into the pulmonary (lung) circulation.

Left heart catheterization is the part of the study that investigates the "left side" of the heart. A specially shaped catheter is inserted into an *artery*, then advanced into the circulation, in a direction opposite to the normal blood flow. The catheter is directed toward the aorta and toward the aortic root (the part of the aorta near the heart). If advanced further, it will go across the aortic valve into the left ventricle. The pressure waves (the "ups and downs" of pressure during the cardiac cycle) are displayed on monitor screens and can be recorded on special tracing paper.

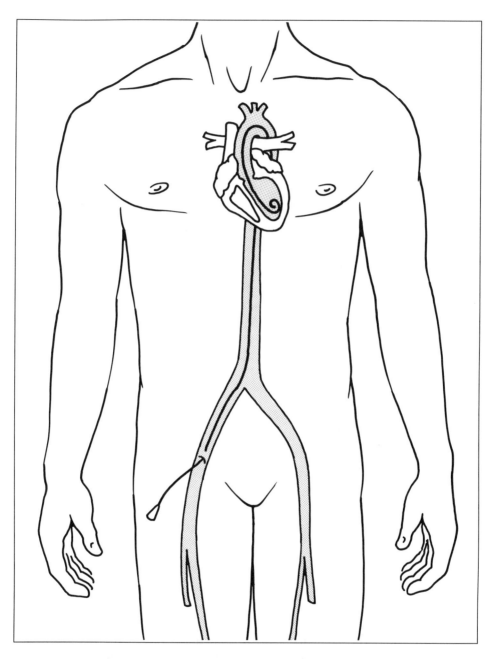

Figure 21. During cardiac catheterization, a catheter is inserted into a peripheral artery (or vein) and then directed toward the heart. Here, the tip of the catheter is shown inside the left ventricle.

During *coronary angiography*, several specially shaped catheters are inserted in sequence into an artery and then directed toward the portion of the aorta near the heart (aortic root) where the coronary arteries originate. Although there are three major coronary arteries, there are only two openings, termed "right" and "left." With x-ray guidance, the cardiologist directs the pre-shaped catheter (either "right" or "left") into the opening of the corresponding coronary artery. When the tip of the catheter is in correct position, dye is injected through the catheter into the coronary artery. (See figure 22). Using a special x-ray movie ("cine") camera, pictures of the coronary arteries are then obtained (the picture is called an angiogram). Multiple "shots" are taken in multiple angles, by tilting the camera (or the table). These multiple views allow a more detailed study of the coronary arteries, and help in detecting areas of narrowing or blockage.

During *left ventricular angiography,* a special catheter with multiple holes near its tip is directed into the aorta and into the left ventricle (the main pumping chamber). After the catheter has been correctly positioned, a larger amount of dye is injected under pressure into the ventricle, and pictures are obtained with the cine camera. The left ventricular angiogram gives a detailed picture of the left ventricle during its contraction and relaxation, and it is particularly useful in assessing the pumping function (contractility) of the heart in various types of heart disease.

A complete cardiac catheterization study (including a coronary angiogram) generally lasts from one to two hours. Patients stay awake during the procedure and are generally able to watch some of the pictures on the television screen. Cardiac catheterization is not an operation. In fact, the patient's cooperation is often needed during the procedure. During the filming of the coronary angiogram, for example, the patient may be asked to take a deep breath and hold it for a few seconds, in order to avoid blurring of the pictures. Other times, he may be asked to cough several times, to help speed the removal of the dye from the coronary arteries.

Cardiac catheterization is not a painful procedure, although some patients may report mild discomfort during the manipulation of the catheters in the groin. Most of the discomfort is generally due to the need to lie still for a prolonged period of time. The advancement of the catheters within the blood vessels and the injection of dye are generally painless. During the injection of dye into the left ventricle, patients may feel a sensation of warmth ("hot flush") all over their body, lasting for about 20 seconds. Some

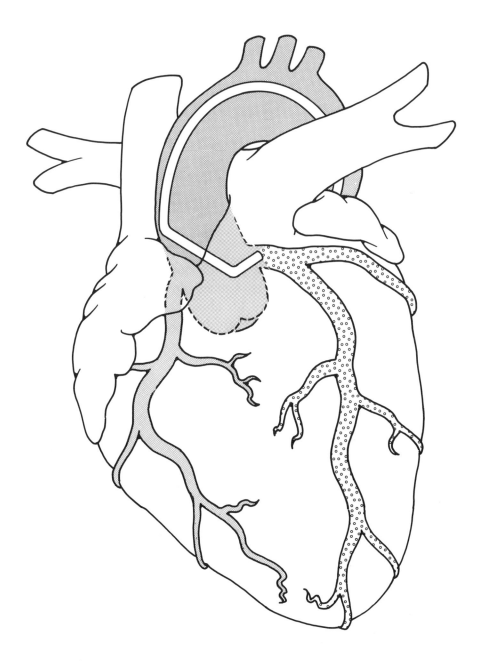

Figure 22. During coronary angiography, a pre-shaped catheter is directed toward the opening of the coronary artery. Dye (contrast) is then injected through the catheter into the artery.

patients may complain of chest discomfort, especially during the injection of dye into the coronary arteries. This sensation is usually temporary, and subsides within a few minutes.

After the Procedure

When the procedure is over, the catheters are pulled out. The physician (or his assistant) applies pressure with a firm hand over the groin area for a period of about 20 minutes, in order to prevent bleeding (if the insertion site was in the arm, the doctor sutures the site of incision with several stitches). The nurse may then apply a weight, usually a 10-pound sand bag, over the catheterization site in the groin. The patient is then gently transferred back to a movable bed, and transported back to his room.

Back in the room, the patient is watched closely for a period of several hours. He will have to lie in bed for about six hours, to assure that no bleeding occurs (if the catheterization site was in the arm, he may be allowed to walk in the room sooner). The nurse will check the blood pressure and pulse frequently, and will also keep checking the site where the catheter was inserted to be sure there is no bleeding.

Most patients resume eating shortly after returning to their room. They are encouraged to drink plenty of water and juices in order to "flush" the dye out of the circulation, and into the urine. About 6 to 8 hours after they have returned to their room, patients are allowed to get out of bed and walk in the room. Patients are generally discharged the morning after the procedure, unless further studies or treatments are indicated.

Possible Risks and Complications

Cardiac catheterization and coronary angiography are "invasive" techniques that require the insertion of catheters and devices that actually enter the body. They are therefore associated with a certain degree of risk. These procedures do not constitute a major operation, however, and the risk is relatively small. Before recommending such procedures, the physician must weigh the benefits to be gained from the study against the possible risks to the patient.

Many of the complications associated with the use of invasive cardiac procedures are considered *minor complications*. They are usually temporary and of no long-term consequence to the patient. Some patients, for example, may develop nausea and vomiting immediately following the injection of dye. Other may develop a reaction to the dye, leading to skin rash (hives), itching, or respiratory distress. The manipulation of catheters within the heart and the injection of dye may result in various cardiac arrhythmias, such as irregular or slow heartbeat. Occasionally, patients may develop bleeding from the catheterization site in the groin. This can be generally controlled by pressing at the site with a firm hand for an extra period of time. In some patients, blood may collect under the skin, resulting in a hematoma, that is, a local swelling or "blue mark" in the groin area. The swelling usually diminishes over a period of several days, and the skin discoloration disappears within a week or two.

Less frequently, invasive cardiac procedures may be associated with *major complications*. The manipulation of catheters inside the blood vessels, for example, may cause vascular damage, and may lead to perforation of the vascular wall or to formation of blood clots. Life-threatening cardiac arrhythmias may occur, requiring prompt treatment. Rarely, a patient may suffer a myocardial infarction (heart attack), either during the procedure or soon after it. Other times, a patient may develop a stroke, generally caused by small blood clots that have traveled from the heart to the brain. Finally, in very rare instances, death can occur, usually the result of a massive heart attack or uncontrollable cardiac arrhythmias.

It should be emphasized, once again, that the risk of sustaining a major complication is relatively small. In patients who are to undergo cardiac catheterization and coronary angiography, the potential risk of suffering a major complication (such as vascular damage, major cardiac arrhythmia, heart attack, or stroke) is approximately 1 to 2 percent. The risk of dying from the procedure is about 0.1 to 0.2 percent. In other words, 1 or 2 out of 100 patients undergoing these procedures may suffer a major complication, and 1 or 2 out of 1000 patients may die from it. This risk may seem high, but it should be remembered that patients who undergo these tests often have significant heart disease to start with, and are therefore at risk of developing problems and complications from their underlying condition unless properly diagnosed and treated!

The Findings Obtained During the Procedure

Following the procedure, it generally takes about an hour or two for the angiogram films to be developed. The various findings (such as the pressure tracings and cine films) are carefully reviewed by the cardiologist. The kind of information looked for in any particular case will vary depending on the nature of the suspected underlying condition. (See figure 23).

The main purpose of cardiac catheterization is the measurement of pressures within the heart chambers and within the major blood vessels (aorta and pulmonary artery). Pressures are obtained by connecting the catheter to a pressure gauge. The pressure of blood at the tip of the catheter is transmitted through the length of the catheter to the pressure gauge. The pressure waves are then displayed on monitoring screens and can be recorded on special tracing paper. Another use of cardiac catheterization is the measurement of the cardiac output, that is, the amount of blood pumped by the heart each minute. The knowledge of the cardiac output is useful for the assessment of the pumping function of the heart in patients with various types of heart disease.

Cardiac catheterization is very useful in the diagnosis of valvular heart disease and congenital heart defects. In patients with a narrowed valve (stenosis), for example, the measurement of the pressures in the various parts of the heart may reveal a difference of pressures (gradient) across the narrowed valve. In patients with a leaky valve (regurgitation), the injection of dye in the appropriate heart chamber or major blood vessel will show abnormal flow of the dye in the "wrong" direction.

Coronary angiography is very useful in the diagnosis of coronary heart disease and angina (see Chapter 13). In fact, it is the only technique that will provide unequivocal diagnostic information regarding the presence or absence of coronary artery disease. In patients with coronary heart disease, the coronary angiogram will show areas of abnormal narrowing or complete obstruction involving one or more of the coronary arteries. The severity of the condition can then be estimated on the basis of several angiographic factors, such as the degree of narrowing, the location of the narrowing(s), and the number of vessels involved. Finally, using the findings on the left ventricular angiogram, the physician can assess the size of the ventricle as well as its contractile (pumping) function.

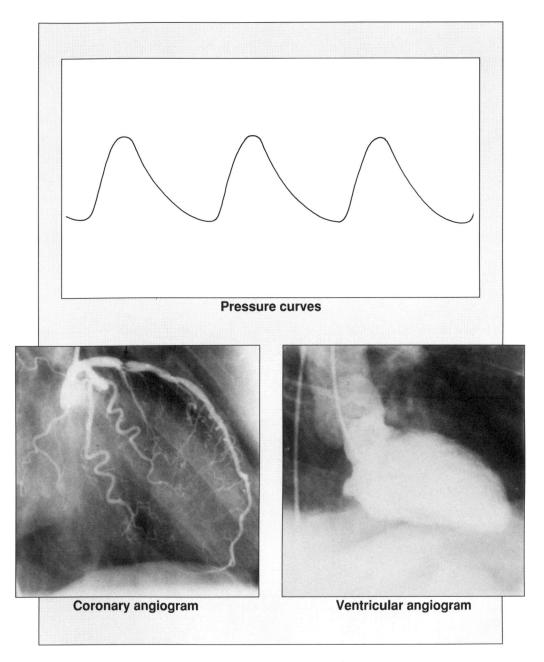

Pressure curves

Coronary angiogram

Ventricular angiogram

Figure 23. The main findings obtained during the cardiac catheterization and angiography procedure include the measurement of pressures within the heart, the coronary angiogram, and the ventricular angiogram.

By combining the information obtained during the procedure with the clinical facts obtained previously (medical history, physical examination, and noninvasive tests), the cardiologist will be able to get an overall picture of the patient's condition. Only then will he be able to make an informed decision regarding the possible approaches to the problem.

At some time prior to discharge from the hospital, the cardiologist will discuss the results with the patient and his family. At that time, he will probably recommend a specific treatment. He may, for example, initiate therapy with cardiovascular drugs. Or, if the problem is serious enough, he may recommend additional therapeutic procedures, such as coronary balloon angioplasty or cardiac surgery. Finally, if the studies show that the condition is mild, he may reassure the patient and advise him to cut down on his cardiac medications.

Part Three

UNDERSTANDING
HEART DISEASE

11 Diseases of the Heart: An Overview

A wide variety of disorders can affect the heart. The mechanism of heart disease is perhaps easier to understand if the heart is likened to a mechanical pump. As we have seen earlier (see Chapter 6), the heart is one of nature's most efficient and durable pumps. Each day it beats more than 100,000 times, and each day it pumps nearly 2000 gallons of blood. The heart works day and night, every day of one's life, and it rests only in between beats, for a split second. But, as with all machines, things can go wrong. . .

Although almost any part of the heart can become defective, the most common problem involves the coronary arteries. Over the years, the inner layer of the arterial wall may become thickened and roughened by deposits of fatty material. The progressive build-up of these fatty deposits causes narrowing of the arterial channel and slowing of the blood flow. *Coronary heart disease* is present when one or more of the coronary arteries are significantly narrowed. In its early stages, coronary heart disease is usually "silent," that is, does not cause any symptoms. With time, however, there is further narrowing of the coronary vessels, eventually leading to serious manifestations, such as angina, heart attack, or sudden death.

In patients with coronary heart disease, the blood flow to the heart muscle is inadequate, and the oxygen supply may not meet the oxygen demand. The imbalance between oxygen supply and demand leads to "starving" of the heart muscle for oxygen, and may result in symptoms of *angina*. Typically, angina is a pressure-like discomfort, located in the middle of the chest, occurring on exertion and relieved at rest, lasting for several minutes. Angina is a warning sign, alerting us to the possibility that there exists a problem with the oxygen supply to the heart muscle.

When one or more of the coronary arteries become severely narrowed by an enlarging plaque, sudden blockage of blood flow may occur, causing the heart muscle to be deprived of oxygen for long periods of time. This may lead to permanent damage to a portion of the heart muscle, a condition termed *heart attack* (or myocardial infarction). The chest pain of a heart attack resembles angina pain in character, but it is much more severe, lasts longer, and does not subside with rest. Heart attack is a serious condition that can lead to severe damage to the heart muscle and to disruption of the cardiac electrical system.

One of the most common medical problems in this country is *high blood pressure* (or hypertension), a condition characterized by an excessive amount of pressure within the arteries. In most patients, the elevated blood pressure produces no symptoms (it is "silent"). If not treated, however, it can lead to progressive damage to the blood vessels and to other vital organs (especially the heart and brain). Although it is not a disease of the heart itself, high blood pressure is one of the three major risk factors for coronary heart disease. Also, the heart suffers from the constant strain of having to pump blood against high resistance. This may lead to weakening of the heart pump and eventually to manifestations of heart failure.

A normal heart valve is flexible enough to open and permit blood to flow through it, yet strong enough to hold back the flow when it is closed. *Valvular heart disease* is present when a heart valve is defective, either "narrowed" or "leaky." A narrowed valve is unable to open fully, thus delaying forward blood flow. A leaky valve, on the other hand, is unable to close completely, thus permitting leakage of blood in the "wrong" direction. Early in the course of the disease, the body itself provides some relief in the form of compensatory mechanisms designed to help the heart pump carry on its function. With time, however, valvular defects tend to get worse, eventually leading to manifestations of heart failure.

When the heart pump becomes too weak, the heart is unable to provide sufficient blood to maintain adequate delivery of oxygen and nutrients to the body tissues. In addition, there is backup of blood in the lungs, resulting in congestion of the lungs. The condition, called *congestive heart failure*, can be caused by a variety of cardiac disorders, such as a previous heart attack, valvular defects (either narrowed or leaky valves), or long-standing high blood pressure. The most common symptom of congestive heart failure is shortness of breath, which results from the congestion of the lungs.

To carry out its task, the heart depends upon the distribution of electrical impulses that travel from the upper chambers (atria) to the pumping chambers (ventricles). Disturbances of the cardiac rhythm, termed *cardiac arrhythmias*, result from disruption in either the formation or the conduction of these electrical impulses. The heart may beat too slowly (bradycardia), too rapidly (tachycardia), or it may become erratic. Patients with cardiac arrhythmias may experience a variety of symptoms, such as palpitations, dizziness, and fainting spells. Most cardiac arrhythmias are temporary and benign; some, however, may be life-threatening.

The development of the fetal heart is a very complex process during which a large number of malformations may occur. *Congenital heart defects* are malformations of the heart that are present at birth. The most common type of congenital defect is due to an abnormal hole in the heart and rerouting of blood flow. Another common type of defect results from an abnormal narrowing of a heart valve and obstruction to blood flow. The defect may be minor, requiring no treatment, or it may be so severe that no effective treatment is available and the infant will die.

12 Coronary Heart Disease

Coronary heart disease is the most common form of heart disease. It is due to the accumulation of fatty deposits in the walls of the coronary arteries, the arteries that feed the heart muscle. The underlying condition, called atherosclerosis, is a degenerative process that involves arteries in the heart, brain, and other parts of the body. The clinical manifestations of coronary heart disease are many, and may include various conditions such as angina, heart attack, and sudden death. Many patients with severe coronary heart disease may be entirely free of symptoms.

Atherosclerosis: The "Silent Disease"

The inside walls of the arteries are normally smooth and flexible, letting the blood flow through them easily. Over the years, the inner layer of the arterial wall may become thickened and roughened by deposits of fat, cholesterol, and cellular debris. This degenerative process, termed atherosclerosis, is the major underlying cause of cardiovascular (pertaining to the heart and blood vessels) diseases. This term should not be confused with arteriosclerosis (commonly called "hardening of the arteries") which is a more general term referring to the hardening and loss of elasticity of the arterial walls associated with the aging process.

As these fatty deposits, called plaques, continue to build up, they project above the surface of the inner layer of the artery, thus decreasing the internal diameter of the blood vessel. (See figure 24). The blood moves with difficulty through the narrowed channel, making it easier for a clot to form,

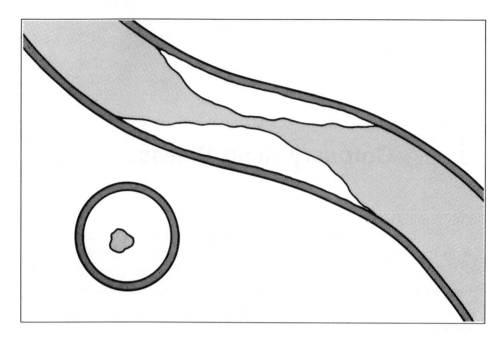

Figure 24. Fatty deposits (plaque) in an artery.

eventually resulting in the complete blockage of the artery. Atherosclerosis most commonly involves the arteries leading to the heart, brain, and lower extremities. When a complete blockage occurs in one of the arteries feeding the heart muscle (coronary arteries) the result is a heart attack. When it occurs in one of the arteries feeding the brain, the result is a stroke.

Atherosclerosis is a slow, progressive disease that begins early in life, as early as childhood and adolescence! It may take years for the plaques to build up enough to slow down the blood flow. In the early stages, the disease is "silent," that is, does not cause any symptoms. The condition is usually not suspected until the arteries are so clogged that a major illness, such as a heart attack or a stroke, results.

There has been a tremendous amount of research done over the past 20 years trying to understand the process of atherosclerosis. It seems, however, that we have just begun to really understand some of its underlying mechanisms. There is strong evidence, for example, that sustained elevation of blood cholesterol can lead to acceleration of the atherosclerotic process. There also exists some connection between the wear and tear of the inner lining of the arteries and the development of plaques. Finally, it has been shown that certain conditions and habits, termed risk factors, do play an important role in the premature development or rapid progression of the disease (see Chapter 2).

Coronary Heart Disease

When atherosclerosis involves the inner walls of the coronary arteries, the result is coronary heart disease. (See figure 25). The progressive build-up of plaques causes narrowing of the arterial channel and thus slowing of the blood flow. The result is inadequate amount of blood and oxygen reaching the heart muscle, leading to "starving" of the heart muscle for oxygen (myocardial ischemia). Further narrowing of the vessel will lead to complete blockage of the artery and permanent damage to the heart muscle (myocardial infarction, or heart attack).

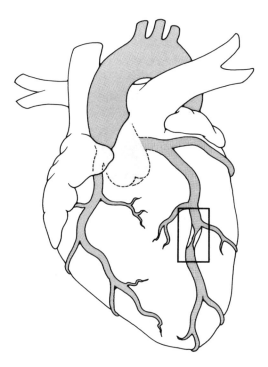

Figure 25. A plaque involving one of the coronary arteries.

Coronary heart disease is the major cause of disability and death in this country. The following facts suggest how much of a problem coronary heart disease is:

- Myocardial infarction (heart attack) is the leading cause of mortality in the United States (550,000 deaths in 1985). It is alone responsible for more deaths each year than all forms of cancer combined.

- As many as 1.5 million Americans will have a heart attack this year alone, and over a third of them will die from it.

- As many as 5 million Americans alive today have a history of heart attack or angina, or both.

- Each year, about 350,000 persons die of a heart attack even before reaching the hospital. The average victim of a heart attack waits three hours before deciding to get help.

- Coronary heart disease often affects people in the prime of life. The average age of men at the time of their first heart attack is in the mid-fifties; for women it is in the mid-sixties.

- The economic cost (health expenditures and lost productivity) attributed to coronary heart disease in 1985 has been estimated at over $50 billion.

. . . .

Coronary heart disease has multiple and varied clinical expressions (see figure 26), which include:

• *Angina:* pain or discomfort in the chest, resulting from inadequate delivery of blood and oxygen to the heart muscle. Angina is often a warning sign in patients with coronary heart disease.

• *Heart attack (or myocardial infarction):* permanent damage to an area of the heart muscle, resulting from a complete blockage of a coronary artery. It is a serious condition, and is often fatal.

• *Non-symptomatic:* many individuals with severe coronary heart disease are entirely free of symptoms. In fact, the first manifestation of the disease is often a heart attack!

• *Congestive heart failure:* the damaged heart muscle is unable to pump sufficient blood to maintain adequate circulation. Heart failure can be caused by a variety of other cardiac conditions.

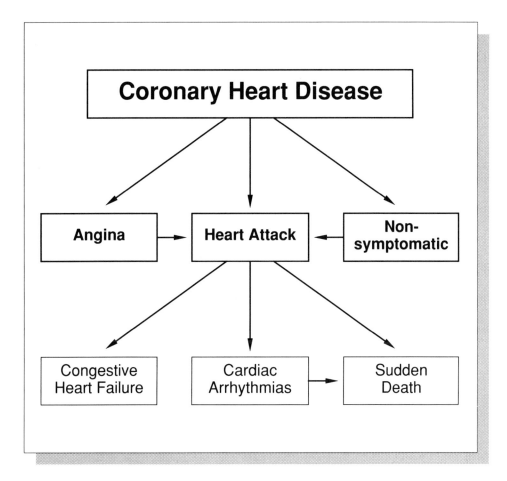

Figure 26. The various manifestations of coronary heart disease.

• *Cardiac arrhythmias:* disturbances in the cardiac rhythm, resulting from disruption of the electrical system of the heart. Many other types of heart disease can lead to cardiac arrhythmias.

• *Sudden death:* may be the first, last, and only manifestation of coronary heart disease. It is usually due to a massive heart attack or a major cardiac arrhythmia. It often occurs without any prior warning.

13 Angina: A Warning Sign

Angina pectoris (or simply angina), a common manifestation of coronary heart disease, is the medical term for pain or discomfort in the chest. Angina results from "starving" of the heart muscle for oxygen (myocardial ischemia), which occurs whenever the heart muscle receives an insufficient supply of blood and oxygen.

Understanding Angina

Coronary heart disease is the result of atherosclerosis, that is, the accumulation of fatty deposits (plaques) inside the coronary arteries. (See Chapter 12). The progressive build-up of plaques on the arterial wall causes narrowing of the channel and slowing of blood flow, and eventually results in an inadequate amount of blood reaching the heart muscle. The narrowing ("lesion") must reduce the diameter of the channel by at least 70% before interfering with the coronary blood flow. In patients with coronary heart disease, symptoms of angina may not occur for years, until the blockage of the artery becomes significant, quite often exceeding 90% narrowing.

Under resting conditions, myocardial oxygen demand and myocardial oxygen supply remain in balance through a complex regulatory mechanism. During exercise activity or emotional upset the heart beats faster and the blood pressure may rise. The heart is performing extra work and thus temporarily needs more oxygen. A normal heart has no problem meeting this extra demand since the coronary arteries are able to deliver enough oxygen to the heart muscle.

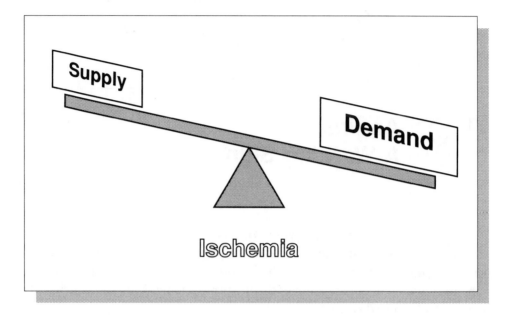

Figure 27. The imbalance between the heart muscle's oxygen supply and demand leads to ischemia.

In patients whose coronary arteries are narrowed at one or more locations, the blood flow to the heart muscle is compromised, and the oxygen supply may not meet the increased demand. (See figure 27). The imbalance between oxygen supply and demand leads to myocardial ischemia ("starving" of the heart muscle for oxygen) and angina. It should be noted, however, that myocardial ischemia does not always result in angina. In fact, it is possible to have significant coronary heart disease and severe ischemia without experiencing any chest pain or discomfort.

In the majority of patients suffering from angina, the narrowing of the coronary arteries is caused by deposits of fatty material. In some patients, however, the narrowing can be caused by a temporary contraction of a segment of the arterial wall, or coronary spasm (see figure 28). Coronary spasm may occur in the absence of any atherosclerotic plaques. In most cases, however, it is superimposed on a pre-existing plaque. In fact, it is now believed that in the majority of patients with symptoms of angina there exists a combination of both a "fixed" narrowing caused by a plaque and an intermittent spasm of the arterial wall.

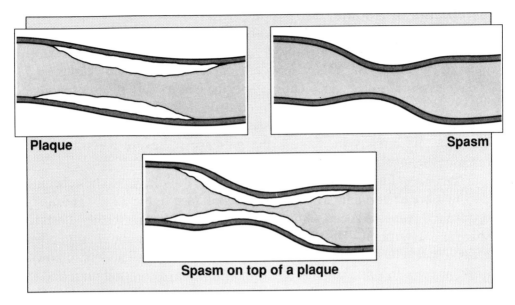

Plaque

Spasm

Spasm on top of a plaque

Figure 28. Coronary spasm is the temporary contraction of a segment of the arterial wall. It is often superimposed on a pre-existing plaque.

Myocardial ischemia is usually a temporary condition that lasts for only a few minutes. However, when one or more of the coronary arteries become severely narrowed by an enlarging plaque or severe spasm (or both), sudden interruption of blood flow may occur. This will cause the heart muscle to be deprived of oxygen for a prolonged period of time, and may result in irreversible damage to the portion of the heart muscle, a condition termed myocardial infarction (or heart attack).

Angina is a warning sign, alerting us to the possibility that a serious problem exists with the oxygen supply to the heart muscle. The presence of angina also informs us that the heart muscle is still alive, and not yet irreversibly damaged. In adults, a new onset of chest pain should never be ignored, because ignoring or denying this important symptom may lead to permanent damage to the heart muscle, and could place one's health and even life in jeopardy.

Symptoms of Angina

Patients with angina often describe their discomfort as a sensation of pressure in the chest. They may use expressions such as "tightness," "heaviness," or "squeezing." Others describe it as a "burning" sensation or "gas," and may mistake it for heartburn or indigestion. Occasionally, angina can be manifested as excessive breathlessness or fatigue during exertion. As already mentioned, the presence of severe coronary heart disease does not always result in symptoms of angina.

The discomfort is most commonly felt in the middle of the chest, behind the breastbone (sternum), or slightly to the left (see figure 29). It is usually diffuse and perceived deep within the chest, although occasionally it can be sharp and superficial. The discomfort often radiates from the chest to other areas, especially the arms (most commonly the left), shoulders, elbows, neck, or jaw. In some patients, the discomfort may be entirely referred to one of these areas in the absence of any discomfort in the chest. For example, it is not unusual for a patient to complain of an isolated "ache" in the shoulder or elbow area. Occasionally, the discomfort may be experienced in the upper abdomen, causing a feeling of "indigestion."

Angina typically occurs during exertion (such as walking fast or climbing stairs), when an extra workload is placed on the heart. The amount of activity required to produce angina may vary among patients. Some activities, such as walking after a heavy meal or against cold wind, often bring on angina at a lower level of activity. In some patients, angina can be precipitated by anger, excitement, or sexual intercourse.

Angina is typically a pain or discomfort of short duration, lasting somewhere between 3 to 15 minutes. It generally subsides soon after the activity has stopped, and there is no residual discomfort. A nitroglycerin pill taken under the tongue will usually relieve the angina episode within less than 3 minutes.

The manifestations of angina differ a great deal among patients. In the individual patient, however, recurrent episodes of angina will usually occur in similar circumstances, and the discomfort will have similar qualities. Patients may have recurrence of angina symptoms for months or even years without any significant change in the pattern. In this type, termed chronic or stable angina, the symptoms remain essentially unchanged in frequency

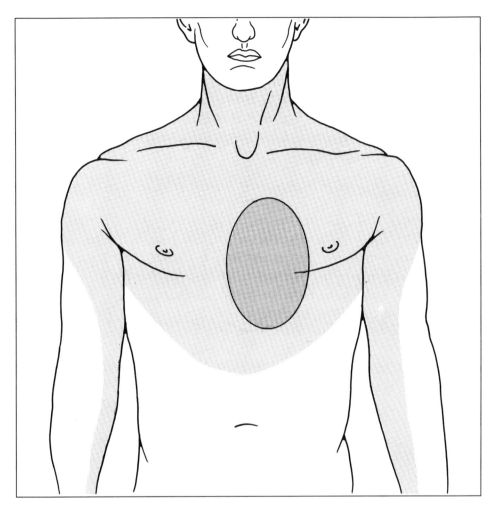

Figure 29. The pain of angina is typically located in the central portion of the chest, and it may radiate to other areas.

and severity, occur at the same level of activity, and are relieved with the same dose of antianginal medications.

It should be emphasized that not every chest pain or discomfort is a manifestation of angina. Pain that mimics angina can arise from other organs within the chest cavity (such as lungs, esophagus, and stomach) or can originate from the bony structures of the chest.

Diagnosing Angina

The diagnosis of angina is generally first considered when an adult patient develops symptoms of chest pain. In fact, a strong presumptive diagnosis of angina can usually be made based on the description of the symptoms alone. Once the diagnosis of angina is suspected, the condition can be assessed with a series of diagnostic tests, such as an exercise stress test and coronary angiography.

Patient History

A thorough medical history generally provides the most useful information for diagnosing angina. The doctor will first listen to the patient's own description of symptoms. The patient may use gestures to characterize the location and quality of his discomfort. Clenching the fist in front of the chest while describing the pressure sensation, for example, is often a good indication for the presence of angina.

The doctor will then ask specific questions regarding the characteristics of the chest discomfort, such as: "What does it feel like?", "Where is it located?", "What brings it on?", and "How long does it usually last?". As we just saw, typical angina is a pressure-like discomfort, located in the middle of the chest, occurring on exertion and relieved at rest, lasting for a period of 3 to 15 minutes.

After reviewing the patient's symptoms, the physician will complete the medical history by asking questions about past and present illnesses, family history, and overall lifestyle. He will especially inquire about the existence of any risk factors, that is, those conditions or habits associated with an increased risk of developing coronary heart disease (such as cigarette smoking, high blood pressure, and high cholesterol level).

Knowledge of the risk factors in the individual patient is helpful in assessing his risk of developing coronary heart disease. However, it is by no means a reliable tool in the diagnosis of angina. As physicians, we sometimes see patients with multiple risk factors who, after an angiogram, are found to have no coronary artery disease. On the other hand, we occasionally see relatively young patients (in their forties and fifties) with no significant risk factors, who develop a major coronary event (such as severe angina or a heart attack).

Exercise Stress Test (Treadmill)

As we just saw, angina results from myocardial ischemia, that is, "starving" of the heart muscle for oxygen. Ischemia occurs whenever the myocardial oxygen supply is unable to meet the increased demand. At rest, the demand is relatively low, and the coronary arteries are able to supply enough oxygen. During exercise activity, however, the heart must perform extra work and thus temporarily needs more oxygen. Since coronary blood flow is already compromised by the narrowing, the oxygen supply becomes insufficient and this may lead to ischemia. An electrocardiogram (ECG) taken during a period of ischemia, will usually (but not always) show abnormal changes, termed "ischemic changes."

A resting ECG (taken under resting conditions) is generally not helpful in diagnosing angina, since the test is normal or nearly so in over half of the patients with chronic (or stable) angina. In fact, many patients suffering from severe angina symptoms during exertion have a perfectly normal tracing at rest.

On the other hand, an ECG taken during an exercise stress test (treadmill) can be very helpful. Most patients with significant narrowing of one or more coronary arteries will display ECG changes during the test, generally in the form of ST segment depression (see figure 19, page 96). If these ECG changes suggest ischemia, especially if they are associated with symptoms of chest pain, the test is considered "positive."

The treadmill stress test is a very helpful diagnostic tool for the assessment of chest pain in adults, especially when the clinical presentation is not entirely typical of angina. Even when the diagnosis of angina appears certain from the patient's description of symptoms, stress testing is frequently used in order to assess the severity of the problem and determine the approach to treatment.

The exercise stress test is not totally reliable, and can sometimes give false results (see page 97). The accuracy of the stress test can be improved by performing a simultaneous thallium scan. Thallium-201 is a radioactive substance picked up by the heart muscle tissue in proportion to the coronary blood flow. During the test, a minute amount of the substance is injected into a vein while the patient exercises. The radioisotope is carried in the bloodstream and diffuses into the heart muscle, preferably into well supplied areas, as opposed to areas with ischemia. Following the exercise, the patient lies down on a table and the imaging process begins using a special gamma camera. The pictures obtained reflect the perfusion (supply) pattern within the heart muscle, with "cold spots" (or perfusion "defects") in areas of ischemia (see figure 20, page 99).

The thallium scan provides very useful information on the location and severity of ischemia . The combination of the ECG stress test with thallium imaging gives an accuracy of approximately 90% in the diagnosis of angina and coronary artery disease. Nevertheless, this technique is expensive and not readily available at all institutions. Its use is best reserved for certain categories of patients such as those who have symptoms of chest pain and a "negative" or non-conclusive ECG stress test.

Coronary Angiography

Coronary angiography is an invasive procedure that provides a detailed picture of the coronary arteries (see Chapter 10). This is the only technique that will provide unequivocal diagnostic information regarding the presence or absence of coronary artery disease. The picture (angiogram) permits estimation of the severity of any narrowing that may be present, with great accuracy. No other test can provide this type of information. Because of its accuracy, coronary angiography is considered the "gold standard" technique in the diagnosis of angina and coronary heart disease.

In patients suspected of having angina and coronary heart disease, a coronary angiogram is useful in answering two important questions:

a) Is there evidence of coronary artery disease? A normal coronary artery has smooth walls and tapers down gradually, giving a certain number of branches. In patients with coronary artery disease, the angiogram shows areas of abnormal narrowing ("lesions") or complete blockage involving the coronary artery or its branches.

b) If coronary artery disease is present, how severe is it? The severity of the problem can be estimated on the basis of several angiographic findings, such as the degree of narrowing, the location of the lesion(s), and the number of blood vessels involved.

A coronary angiogram is often recommended in patients with unexplained symptoms of chest pain in whom the exercise stress test is non-conclusive, and in patients with multiple hospital admissions for a possible heart attack when the diagnosis has never been substantiated. In such individuals, a normal coronary angiogram may help reassure the patient (as well as his physician) and may prevent undue anxiety as well as unnecessary hospitalizations and expenses.

Despite its accuracy and usefulness, a coronary angiogram cannot be recommended to every patient suspected of having angina. First, it is an expensive test, and patients have to be hospitalized. Second, it is an invasive procedure, requiring insertion of a catheter which actually enters the body, and it therefore entails a certain degree of risk. It should be emphasized, however, that the angiogram is not considered a major surgical procedure, and the risk is relatively small. Before recommending a coronary angiogram, the cardiologist must weigh the benefits to be gained from the procedure against the possible risks to the patient.

The Management of Angina

There are several goals in managing patients with chronic "stable" angina. The first goal is to prevent symptoms, or at least significantly reduce the frequency and severity of angina attacks. The second objective is to enable these patients to maintain their accustomed lifestyle. Too many patients "live with" angina by severely limiting their activities. They know which activities bring on their attacks, so they simply avoid them. In this way they stop getting symptoms, but also give up many important aspects of their lives. Finally, the third goal is to prolong the life of these patients by preventing the occurrence of a heart attack and premature death.

General Measures

Effective communication between the physician and the patient is essential to good medical management. Too many patients have an unrealistically gloomy perception of their disease. The physician's role is to provide an understandable explanation of the clinical features together with a realistic appraisal of the disease. Reassurance is important: the patient must realize that an active and useful life is possible even though he has angina. Another important aspect of the physician's role is to counsel patients regarding the kind of work they do, their leisure activities, eating habits, vacation plans, and so on.

In some patients, certain changes in lifestyle will be necessary. Certain strenuous activities may have to be modified if they constantly and repeatedly produce angina. For example, a golfer complaining of recurrent angina on the golf course might use a golf cart instead of walking. Many activities such as shopping or climbing stairs need not be discontinued. Often it is merely necessary to perform them more slowly, or pause for brief periods of rest.

Patients must avoid excessive fatigue and exhaustion. One or two regular rest periods during each day are particularly helpful. As a rule of thumb, the stress of sexual intercourse is approximately equal to that of an exercise that induces a heart rate of 120 per minute. With proper precautions, the majority of patients with chronic angina will be able to continue a satisfactory sex life.

As we have seen, certain habits or conditions, termed risk factors, are associated with an increased risk of developing coronary heart disease. Therefore, it seems reasonable to modify these risk factors in order to slow down the progression of the disease. Patients with angina should:

- Give up cigarette smoking
- Eat a proper diet, low in fat and cholesterol
- Maintain a desirable body weight
- Exercise regularly

Patients with chronic angina should be encouraged to engage in a regular exercise program, such as walking, jogging, biking, or swimming. Regular exercise has a beneficial conditioning effect on the heart muscle. Patients involved in an exercise program are more apt to be health conscious, to pay attention to diet and weight, and to give up smoking. In addition, regular exercise provides the individual with a feeling of well-being. Any exercise program in patients with angina should be supervised, at least initially. An exercise stress test is useful both to evaluate the safety of and to determine reasonable limits for the exercise activity.

Drug Therapy

As discussed above, angina is the result of myocardial ischemia, which occurs whenever the heart muscle's available oxygen supply does not meet its oxygen demand. In general terms, the treatment of angina can be aimed either at reducing the oxygen requirements of the heart muscle or at increasing the coronary blood flow.

The three major classes of antianginal drugs available today are the nitrates, the beta blockers, and the calcium channel blockers. By their action, these agents can favorably affect the imbalance between the myocardial oxygen demand and supply, and thus relieve or prevent angina attacks. When properly selected, these medications are capable of providing good control of symptoms as well as improvement in exercise tolerance in the majority of patients.

The Nitrates. The nitrates are vasodilator drugs: they relax the walls of blood vessels, both veins and arteries, causing them to dilate. They exert a beneficial influence by decreasing myocardial oxygen demand and by increasing blood supply to ischemic areas.

The nitrates reduce myocardial oxygen demand indirectly by two different mechanisms. First, they dilate the veins throughout the body, causing them to retain more blood, which would normally go to the heart. Thus, less blood returns to the heart, and less blood has to be pumped by the left ventricle (the main pumping chamber). As a result, the heart has less work to perform and therefore needs less oxygen. In addition, the nitrates cause dilatation of the arteries throughout the body, thus lowering the resistance against which the left ventricle must pump during its contraction, resulting once again in less workload and therefore decreased myocardial oxygen demand.

On the supply side, nitrates increase the blood flow to the heart muscle by two mechanisms. First, they dilate the coronary arteries, even in areas of severe fixed narrowing. In addition, they relieve or prevent coronary spasm, regardless of whether it is isolated or superimposed on a pre-existing "fixed" coronary lesion.

Nitroglycerin remains the most effective drug for the relief of an angina attack. During an episode of angina, the tiny nitroglycerin tablet is placed under the tongue and allowed to dissolve, often giving a slight tingling sensation. The angina pain is usually relieved within a few minutes. Nitroglycerin is a short-acting drug which does not accumulate in the body. Therefore, it may be taken repeatedly without becoming ineffective or habit forming. It should be emphasized, however, that if the pain does not subside or if it becomes worse, the patient should seek medical help, because the symptoms may be a manifestation of an impending heart attack.

Nitroglycerin can also be used before symptoms occur, in anticipation of activities or situations that usually bring on angina, such as strenuous physical activity, sexual intercourse, or emotional stress. Some patients, for example, are prone to develop angina during the one-hour period following a heavy meal. Taking a nitroglycerin tablet at the end of the meal might get these patients safely through that period without getting symptoms.

In addition to the short-acting nitroglycerin preparations, there are several long-acting nitrates, used for the prevention of angina attacks. These preparations are ineffective in relieving angina once it has occurred, but are useful in preventing the onset of symptoms. They are administered several times a day depending upon their duration of action. The oral preparations (tablets and capsules), for example, are usually taken 4 times a day. Nitroglycerin is also available in ointment form, which is applied to the skin (most commonly on the chest) 3 or 4 times a day.

Recently, transdermal patches have made the delivery of nitroglycerin more convenient and less messy. The patch is applied to the skin once a day, and nitroglycerin gradually diffuses through the skin at a constant rate over a period of 24 hours.

Nitrates are generally safe and well tolerated. The most common troubling side effect is headache. It is often possible to eliminate or minimize the headache by starting with small dosages and slowly working up to effective dosages, or by taking a pain medication to relieve the headache. Other side effects that may occur with the use of nitrates are dizziness, palpitations, and low blood pressure.

The Beta Blockers. Unlike the nitrates which act by affecting the peripheral blood vessels, the beta blockers act upon the heart muscle directly. These drugs block the action of the beta receptors, that is, the nerve endings that affect the heart rate and force of contraction (contractility). As a result, they reduce the amount of work performed by the heart, and thus reduce the myocardial oxygen demand.

During physical activity or emotional stress, there is normally an increase of both heart rate and contractility. In patients taking beta blockers the rise in these two parameters is slower, and myocardial oxygen requirements are thereby lower at any given level of activity. This explains why angina patients taking beta blockers are able to exercise for longer periods of time without getting symptoms.

Beta blockers are generally given together with nitrates. This combination is quite effective in the treatment of angina. Currently there are about a dozen different beta blockers available, mostly in tablet form. These are all effective agents, and none seems to have definite superiority over the others. Some of the newer drugs have additional pharmacological properties that may render them more advantageous for specific patients. For example, some have a longer duration of action, and can be taken once a day instead of three or four times a day. Besides their effectiveness in relieving angina symptoms, the beta blockers are also useful in the treatment of other forms of heart disease, such as high blood pressure and the control of certain cardiac arrhythmias.

The beta blockers are generally well tolerated; nevertheless, certain adverse reactions can result from their use. When given to patients whose heart function is severely affected, they may precipitate heart failure, since they reduce the contractility of the left ventricle (the main pumping chamber). In patients with chronic lung disease or asthma, they may cause shortness of breath and wheezing to worsen. The beta blockers cause slowing of the heart rate in almost all patients. If an overly large dose is taken, however, they may cause an excessive slowing of the heart beat, occasionally resulting in symptoms of dizziness and fatigue.

There have been reports of increased anginal symptoms and heart attacks following abrupt discontinuation of beta blockers in patients on long-term therapy. For this reason, patients should never stop taking the beta blockers abruptly and without their physician's knowledge.

The Calcium Channel Blockers. The calcium channel blockers block the transport of calcium in blood vessels and heart muscle cells. Vascular smooth muscle cells (present in the walls of arteries and veins) and heart muscle cells require the presence of intracellular calcium ions in order to contract. Extracellular calcium is actively transported across the muscle cell wall into the interior of the cell through a special "channel." If this calcium transport is blocked, vascular and cardiac muscle contraction is partially inhibited.

By their action, the calcium channel blockers relax the walls of the coronary arteries, and thus prevent coronary spasm. In addition, like the nitrates, they relax the walls of the peripheral blood vessels, lowering the resistance against which the left ventricle must pump, thus resulting in less workload on the heart. By acting directly on the heart muscle, these agents also cause a slight decrease of myocardial contractility, thus further reducing oxygen requirements. The net results of these multiple actions is an increase of coronary blood supply and a reduction in myocardial oxygen demand, both beneficial effects in patients with angina.

Because of their ability to relax the coronary arteries, the calcium channel blockers are very effective in the treatment and prevention of coronary spasm. They are also effective in the management of patients with chronic stable angina, especially those who continue having symptoms despite optimal doses of nitrates and beta blockers.

Three calcium channel blockers are currently available in the United States (nifedipine, verapamil, and diltiazem). They are available as oral preparations (tablets or capsules), and are usually taken 3 or 4 times a day. The various calcium channel blockers are generally well tolerated, and differ to some extent in the type and incidence of side effects. Reported side effects include hypotension (low blood pressure), cardiac arrhythmias, dizziness, headaches, leg swelling, and constipation.

Coronary Balloon Angioplasty

The technique of coronary balloon angioplasty (also termed Percutaneous Transluminal Coronary Angioplasty, or PTCA) is a procedure used to dilate the coronary arteries at the point where they have become narrowed by a plaque. This relatively new technique was introduced in the late 1970s, and promises to be an effective alternative to coronary bypass surgery in carefully selected patients.

During the angioplasty procedure, a special catheter with a tiny balloon at its tip is passed through an artery in the leg or arm and guided into the diseased coronary artery. When the balloon reaches the narrowed portion of the artery, it is inflated several times, thus compressing the plaque against the walls of the artery. When the balloon is withdrawn, the plaque remains compressed, therefore improving the coronary blood flow to the heart muscle (for a more complete discussion, see Chapter 23).

Patient selection for coronary balloon angioplasty is based on the clinical manifestations and the results of the coronary angiogram. The "ideal" candidate for coronary angioplasty is a patient with disabling angina, whose angiogram reveals an isolated distinct narrowing involving the proximal (near the origin) portion of a single coronary artery. Since its introduction in the late 1970s, however, the technique has been constantly refined and patient selection criteria have expanded. Today, for example, coronary angioplasty is often performed in patients with more than one narrowing in a single vessel, or in those with several distinct narrowings in more than one vessel.

When feasible, coronary balloon angioplasty has a number of advantages over bypass surgery. First, it is a relatively brief procedure, which does not necessitate general anesthesia and does not require surgical opening of the chest. In addition, the procedure is less costly, hospitalization is shorter, and the return to work more rapid. It is important to emphasize, however, that this technique has several technical limitations and thus cannot always replace bypass surgery. At the present time, approximately 30 percent of patients who are candidates for surgery can benefit from this less invasive procedure.

Coronary Bypass Surgery

The purpose of coronary bypass surgery is to restore the flow of blood to areas of the heart muscle that receive an inadequate amount of oxygen as a result of narrowed or blocked coronary arteries. The objective of surgery is not to remove the narrowed portion of the artery or the blockage, but rather to create a "bypass" that lets the blood go around it.

To accomplish a bypass, a segment of saphenous vein from the leg is removed to be used as a vein graft. The vein is then attached at one end to a small opening made in the aorta (the body's main artery) and the other end is sewn to an opening created in the coronary artery, beyond the narrowing or blockage (for further discussion, see Chapter 24).

Since it was introduced in the late 1960s, coronary bypass surgery has gained increasing popularity as a therapeutic option for patients with angina and severe coronary artery disease. Over the past decade or two, the procedure has become more refined, both in terms of patient selection and operative techniques. The rates of mortality and morbidity associated with the operation have dropped significantly, especially with the more experienced surgical teams.

There is still considerable controversy among physicians regarding the specific indications for bypass surgery. Despite several large scale studies performed over the past decade, there is still no specific formula upon which all physicians agree that will clearly determine who is a candidate for the surgery and who is not.

Two major factors are usually considered in arriving at a decision whether to advise a coronary bypass operation: a) the severity of angina symptoms and the degree of disability; and b) the number, location, and severity of the coronary lesions as demonstrated by coronary angiography.

Based on the above information, it is then possible to define two general subgroups of patients who will most likely benefit from bypass surgery:

• Patients with persistent disabling symptoms of angina despite optimal doses of antianginal medications.

• The presence of a significant narrowing of the left main coronary artery (before it divides into the two left coronary arteries), or the presence of severe narrowing in at least two of the three major coronary arteries. Since the life expectancy of these patients can often be prolonged with surgery, they should be considered as potential candidates even if their symptoms can be controlled with medications.

In some patients the indications for bypass surgery is far from clear-cut, and the decision whether to operate or not may be difficult. In such patients, the decision process should involve combined efforts of the primary care physician (internist or family practitioner), the cardiologist, and the cardiac surgeon. The potential benefits from the surgery should be weighed against the possible risks, and the various options (if available) should be clearly presented to the patient and his family.

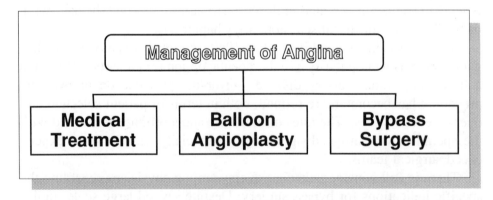

Figure 30. Treatment options in patients with angina.

Unstable Angina

In its most common presentation, angina has a "stable" pattern: symptoms remain basically unchanged in frequency and severity over a period of months or years, and occur at a predictable level of activity. In some patients, however, there may be a noticeable change in the pattern of "their" angina, over a period of weeks, days, or hours. This presentation, termed "unstable" angina, is a serious condition, since it generally indicates a critically compromised coronary circulation.

Symptoms of unstable angina can appear in one of several ways. Some patients may complain of recent onset (less than a month) of angina during exertion. Others may develop a changing pattern or progression of previously "stable" angina. This may include increased frequency or severity of pain with the same activity; angina at a lower level of exercise; or decreased responsiveness to nitroglycerin. Finally, some patients may complain of angina symptoms at rest (driving, eating, watching television, etc.) or during sleep.

Unstable angina is a potentially serious condition. It generally indicates that the coronary circulation is severely compromised, and that there is a critical narrowing of at least one of the three major coronary arteries. Unstable angina is often an indication of an impending myocardial infarction (heart attack). In fact, the term "pre-infarction angina" has often been used by doctors to define the condition in patients with typical symptoms of unstable angina. Studies have shown that among patients admitted to the hospital with symptoms of unstable angina, as many as 30 percent will suffer a heart attack within the ensuing 3-month period.

Patients with unstable angina should be hospitalized, preferably in a coronary care unit, where they can be observed and managed until their symptoms subside. Serial ECGs will be performed and blood samples will be drawn, in order to "rule out" the presence of a myocardial infarction. Medical management usually includes bed rest, sedation, oxygen, and various medications. Drugs used in the control of unstable angina include nitrates, beta blockers, and calcium channel blockers. The symptoms of the majority of patients with unstable angina will be controlled, at least initially, with medical treatment.

Patients who continue to have recurrent chest pain despite vigorous medical treatment are at high risk of myocardial infarction or death. In this

Remember!

Notify your doctor without delay if there has been a noticeable change in the pattern of "your" angina:
- The pain or discomfort is more severe than usual
- It lasts for longer periods of time
- It occurs at more frequent intervals
- It is brought on by a lesser amount of activity
- It is not helped with the usual dose of nitroglycerin

group of patients, a coronary angiogram is usually recommended as early as possible, to determine accurately the extent of the disease, and for consideration of an emergency surgical procedure (coronary bypass surgery or balloon angioplasty).

Some of those who respond favorably to the initial medical management will continue to be pain-free for a while. A larger number of patients, however, will develop either disabling exertional angina with activity or recurrent unstable angina. For this reason, a coronary angiogram is now recommended in most patients with unstable angina.

The coronary angiogram will, first of all, help identify high-risk patients with left main or three-vessel coronary artery disease, in whom surgery is generally helpful in controlling angina and prolonging life. In some, the coronary angiogram will reveal a lesser degree of disease, perhaps a narrowing involving one major coronary artery. Some of these patients may be candidates for coronary balloon angioplasty. In other patients, the angiogram may show only mild disease, without any "threatening" coronary narrowings. Many of these patients will be advised to continue or reduce their antianginal medications. Finally, in a number of patients, the coronary angiogram will reveal normal or minimally diseased coronary arteries. These patients will be reassured and probably advised to cut down on their antianginal medications.

14 Heart Attack

Myocardial infarction (or simply "M.I."), the medical term for a heart attack, is one of a number of possible manifestations of coronary heart disease (see Chapter 12). It is the irreversible damage (infarction) to an area of the heart muscle (myocardium) caused by a total blockage of a coronary artery. It is the end result of the slow degenerative process, called atherosclerosis, involving the coronary arteries.

Myocardial infarction is the leading cause of death in this country and other industrialized nations. It alone is responsible for more deaths than all forms of cancer combined. As many as 1.5 million Americans will have a heart attack this year alone, and over one third of them will die from it. Myocardial infarction often affects men and women in their prime of life. In fact, the average age at the time of their first heart attack is the mid-fifties for men, the mid-sixties for women.

Understanding Myocardial Infarction

During the process of atherosclerosis, which begins early in life and progresses over a period of years, the inner layer of the arteries becomes thickened and roughened by deposits of fat, cholesterol, and cellular debris. As these deposits, called plaques, continue to build up, the inside of the artery becomes narrowed, thus causing restriction of blood flow to the heart muscle. When one or more of the coronary arteries become severely narrowed by an enlarging plaque, sudden blockage of blood flow may occur, causing the heart muscle to be deprived of oxygen for long periods of time. This eventually leads to the irreversible damage and death of the portion of heart muscle supplied by that artery.

Although there still exists some controversy among researchers regarding the exact cause for the sudden blockage, it is believed that three major mechanisms are involved:

a) The enlarging plaque itself can cause critical narrowing of the artery, producing severe and prolonged myocardial ischemia ("starving" of the heart muscle for oxygen), which in turn can result in irreversible damage to the heart muscle.

b) A blood clot (thrombus) often forms in the narrowed portion of the artery, resulting in the sudden "sealing off" of the vessel (figure 31).

c) In some cases, a prolonged spasm (contraction of a segment of the artery) superimposed on the plaque interrupts the blood flow long enough to cause damage to the heart muscle.

The location and the extent of the damage done to the heart muscle depends primarily on the specific coronary artery involved and its relative size. (See figure 32). Blockage of the left anterior descending artery, for example, will cause an infarction of the anterior wall, or the "front" part of the left ventricle (the main pumping chamber). Obstruction of the right coronary artery will result in damage to the inferior wall, or "back" part of the ventricle. Blockage of the circumflex artery will result in damage to the lateral wall, or "side" part of the ventricle. When the obstruction involves

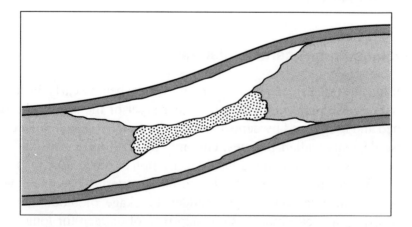

Figure 31. During a heart attack, there is often formation of a fresh blood clot in the narrowed portion of the artery.

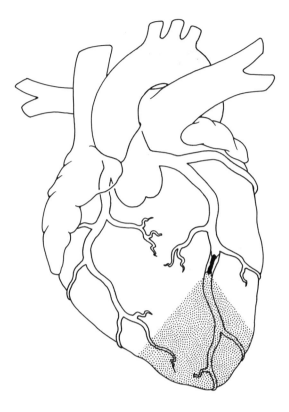

Figure 32. The blockage of a coronary artery causes irreversible damage (infarction) to a functioning segment of the heart muscle.

the left main coronary artery (before it divides into the two left branches), the result is usually a massive myocardial infarction, often leading to irreversible shock and death of the patient.

The primary consequence of the myocardial infarction is the loss of a functioning segment of the heart muscle. In general terms, when the damage involves an area that is more than 30 percent of the left ventricular heart muscle, it often results in manifestations of congestive heart failure. When the damaged area exceeds 50 percent of the ventricle, it usually leads to severe "pump failure" which is fatal in most cases. The infarction may also cause disruption of the electrical system of the heart, leading to disturbances of the cardiac rhythm (cardiac arrhythmias) which may be quite serious and even life-threatening if not treated promptly.

Initial manifestations of the M.I.

Chest pain is the most common initial symptom in patients with acute ("fresh") myocardial infarction. In some instances, the pain may be severe enough to be described as the worst pain the patient has ever experienced. The pain of myocardial infarction resembles angina pain in quality, but is more severe, lasts much longer, and does not disappear with rest.

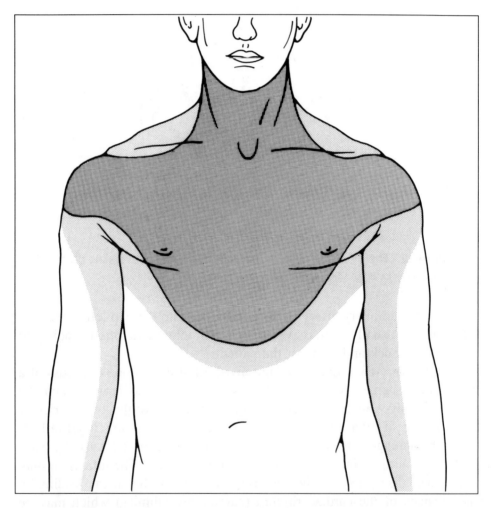

Figure 33. The pain of a heart attack is typically located in the central portion of the chest, and it may radiate to other areas. It resembles angina pain in quality, but is more severe and lasts longer.

The pain of a heart attack is often described as "a heavy weight," "squeezing," or "crushing." It is typically located in the central portion of the chest, under the breastbone, and it may radiate to other areas such as the arms, jaw, neck, or shoulders (see figure 33). The pain is often unbearable and is not relieved by nitroglycerin tablets or by any of the other antianginal medications. It may last for several hours until relieved by narcotic medications (such as morphine) injected into the vein.

Patients having a myocardial infarction often break out in a cold sweat, feel weak and apprehensive, complain of shortness of breath, nausea and vomiting, or "gas" pain. In some patients the pain or discomfort is located in the upper abdomen, and it may be easily mistaken for "indigestion."

Although chest pain is the most common complaint, it is by no means always present. In fact, as many as 15 percent of infarctions are painless! The incidence of painless infarctions is greater in patients with diabetes and in the elderly. Not infrequently, a person is informed that he has had a past infarction (after an ECG) of which he was never aware. This happens when the pain was so mild that the symptoms were ignored or were attributed to a familiar discomfort such as indigestion, and quickly dismissed.

Remember!

When you suffer a heart attack, every minute counts. Do not ignore the warning signals, hoping that they will somehow disappear. Get help immediately. Although the initial symptoms of a heart attack are not the same for every victim, the usual warning signals include:

• Uncomfortable chest pain or discomfort, often described as "pressure," "heavy weight," "squeezing," or "crushing."

• The pain is typically in the center of the chest, behind the breastbone. It may spread to other sites, such as the upper abdomen, shoulders, arms, neck, or jaw.

• The pain may be mistaken for "gas" or "indigestion."

• The pain is often accompanied by a cold sweat, weakness, nausea, vomiting, dizziness, shortness of breath, or marked anxiety.

Diagnosing the M.I.

The diagnosis of myocardial infarction is often suspected on the basis of the presenting symptoms alone. Once an M.I. is suspected, the patient is generally hospitalized, and a series of tests are performed to either confirm or rule out the diagnosis. The two most helpful laboratory tests are the electrocardiogram (ECG) and the measurement of cardiac enzymes.

During the initial few hours following the onset of symptoms, the diagnosis of myocardial infarction can be difficult, since the initial symptoms can be mild or nonspecific. The initial ECG done in the doctor's office or in the emergency room may not be of any help, since it can be perfectly normal! Great skill and good clinical judgment are often required by the physician to be able to distinguish between medical emergencies, such as myocardial infarction or unstable angina, and other less urgent medical conditions.

Even when the initial symptoms are not quite typical, it is often wise to keep the patient in the hospital. In fact, "missing" the diagnosis and discharging the patient home could be of serious consequence. For this reason, most patients will be admitted for observation, for a period of 24 to 48 hours. The admitting diagnosis in such patients is termed "Rule Out M.I.," meaning that the diagnosis of myocardial infarction is suspected but is not definite, and additional diagnostic tests are necessary.

The Electrocardiogram (ECG)

The acute M.I. produces a series of abnormalities that can be detected on the standard resting electrocardiogram (ECG). (See Chapter 9). These abnormalities represent changes of the electrical currents within the heart, resulting from the injury to the heart muscle. The characteristic pattern consists of specific changes that evolve over a period of hours and days. By observing the infarction pattern in specific leads of the ECG, the doctor is able to specify which areas of the ventricular wall have been damaged.

At the onset, there is typically an elevation of the ST segment (the portion between the QRS complex and the T wave), representing "injury" to the heart muscle in the area immediately surrounding the infarction (see figure 34). Several hours later an abnormal Q wave appears, representing the "infarction" area itself. Over the following hours and days, there is a progressive return of the ST segment to the baseline, but with persistence of the abnormal Q wave. Since they represent dead scar tissue, these Q waves will persist indefinitely. In fact, their presence on an ECG is usually a sign that the person has had a heart attack sometime in the past.

Measurements of Cardiac Enzymes

When the heart muscle cells are irreversibly injured during a myocardial infarction, a number of enzymes are released into the circulation. These enzymes are complex molecules that are normally involved in the metabolic functions of the heart muscle cells. They escape from the heart into the bloodstream when the cells die. Following the infarction, there is an abnormal rise in the activity level of these enzymes in the blood, and this can be detected through analysis of blood samples during the first few days following the infarction. (See figure 34).

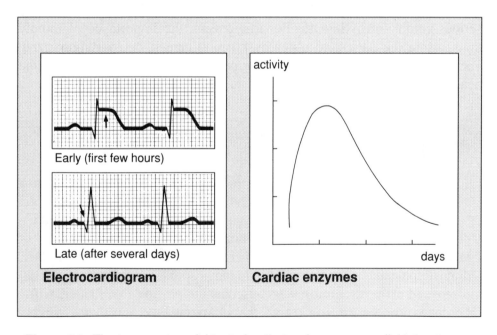

Figure 34. The two most useful tests for diagnosing a myocardial infarction are the electrocardiogram and the measurement of cardiac enzymes.

Management of the M.I.

Over half of the deaths associated with myocardial infarction occur within the first two hours after the onset of symptoms! These early deaths usually result from serious cardiac arrhythmias (disturbances of the cardiac rhythm). Careful monitoring of the cardiac rhythm and prompt treatment of arrhythmias have sharply reduced the incidence of death among hospitalized patients. Indeed, the reduction of the in-hospital mortality from 30 to 15 percent can be attributed to the use of special measures such as the rapid transfer of patients with a suspected heart attack to specialized facilities. These modern facilities are equipped with ECG monitoring capabilities, and are staffed with personnel knowledgeable in the recognition and management of cardiac arrhythmias and other cardiac emergencies.

The Importance of Early Hospitalization

As we have seen, most deaths associated with a heart attack occur within the first two hours after the onset of symptoms, and are usually due to serious cardiac arrhythmias. For this reason, the importance of rapidly transporting the patient to a nearby hospital cannot be overemphasized. Well-equipped ambulances, staffed by personnel trained in the care of the heart attack victim, allow treatment to start while the patient is being

---

Remember!

If you feel you may be having a heart attack, make immediate arrangements to be transported to a hospital emergency room. Do not spend time trying to reach a physician. Call the local emergency number, an ambulance service, or a taxicab. If the hospital is close by, you may let a bystander drive you there. Remember: no harm will be done if you make an occasional trip to the hospital emergency room and discover that the discomfort was caused by indigestion. Much harm will be done, however, if you ignore the symptoms and stay home while having a heart attack!

transported to the hospital. Some of these modern ambulances, called "mobile coronary care units," are equipped with ECG monitoring devices, oxygen, resuscitation equipment, battery-operated defibrillator, and commonly used cardiac drugs.

All too often, the biggest delay is not the time period of transportation to the hospital, but rather the time elapsed between the onset of symptoms (chest pain) and the patient's decision to call for help. In fact, heart attack victims wait an average of three hours before deciding to seek medical help! It is hoped that the delay can be reduced by educating the public about the significance of chest pain and the importance of seeking medical care as early as possible.

The Coronary Care Unit (CCU)

The Coronary Care Unit is a specially designed nursing unit, staffed with trained nursing personnel who have the authority to take immediate action in emergency situations. The CCU allows continuous monitoring of the cardiac rhythm by highly trained nurses who are authorized to administer emergency treatment even in the absence of the physician. Although a physician is available at all times, many lives have been saved because nurses have treated life-threatening cardiac arrhythmias before the physician arrived.

Most patients with a "fresh" heart attack are admitted to a CCU, where they can be observed closely during the initial and critical phase (generally 3 to 4 days). The typical CCU is formed of 6 to 10 small-size rooms, encircling a central monitoring station, where nurses can watch the patient's ECG rhythm 24 hours a day. Glass walls permit the nurse at the central station to watch the patients. The room itself is equipped with a small monitor screen that displays the patient's ECG and pulse rate, oxygen outlets, and various resuscitation equipment.

On his arrival at the CCU, electrodes are attached to the patient's chest, so that his heart rhythm can be constantly monitored. An intravenous line is inserted into a peripheral vein in the arm, and kept open by a slow infusion of glucose (sugar) solution. This open line allows administration of drugs directly into the vein in case of major cardiac arrhythmias or other emergency situations. The patient is also given oxygen-enriched air for inhalation, either through an oxygen face mask or a nasal tubing.

Management of the non-complicated M.I.

The two primary objectives of the initial management in patients with myocardial infarction are:

a) Prevent death from cardiac arrhythmias.

b) Minimize the extent of damage to the heart muscle.

These two objectives are best met in a CCU setting. Patients are monitored constantly, and cardiac arrhythmias can be treated promptly by trained nurses, using the appropriate equipment. To minimize the extent of damage to the heart muscle, the patient is initially maintained at bed rest, given medications for pain relief, and kept under mild sedation in a quiet and restful atmosphere.

During the first few hours after a myocardial infarction, most patients complain of severe chest pain. If not relieved promptly, the severe discomfort can cause significant anxiety, restlessness, and increased heart rate, all of which can result in a detrimental rise in the heart's workload. Pain relief is therefore one of the most important therapeutic objectives in patients with a heart attack. Morphine, which is a potent narcotic, is the drug of choice in treating severe chest pain, and it is most effective when given directly into the vein.

Most patients admitted to the CCU are initially apprehensive and anxious, and some may have a feeling of impending doom. Mild sedation with oral medications is often effective in reducing that anxiety, and it also makes it easier for the patient to cope with the long period of imposed inactivity. Appropriate medication may be given at night to ensure adequate sleep. The role of the CCU nurse is very important in creating a peaceful and reassuring atmosphere, and in encouraging the patient during the initial period of recovery.

During the first day or two, the diet is usually soft, low in fat, and easily digestible. Coffee is best avoided at this stage, since it may induce acceleration of the heart rate and cardiac arrhythmias. As the patient's condition improves and his appetite increases, a more liberal diet is allowed. Bed rest for several days often leads to mild constipation, and this can be often improved by the routine prescription of a stool softener or a mild laxative. Since attempts to use a bed pan often result in excessive straining, most doctors will allow their patients to use a bedside commode.

Activity and Hospital Course

The healing process, during which scar tissue replaces the damaged heart muscle, requires several weeks. During that period, factors that increase the workload on the heart may increase the size of the infarction. The purpose of reduced physical activity during the period of recovery is to provide the most favorable circumstances for the healing process. The purpose of a gradual progression of activity, on the other hand, is to counteract the weakening effect of rest and inactivity.

The patient with a heart attack is generally admitted to the CCU, and usually stays there for 3 to 4 days. During the first 2 or 3 days, he will remain in bed rest most of the day with one or two brief periods of sitting in a bedside chair. The patient may use a bedside commode, and may be bathed by a nurse. He is then encouraged to help himself with feeding, shaving, and bathing.

On the third or fourth day, patients are transferred to the Intermediate Care Unit. By this time most patients will be spending up to an hour in a chair, several times a day. If recovery continues without incident, limited ambulation (walking) within the room is begun somewhere between the fourth and seventh days. Patients can walk around while under continuous ECG monitoring with the aid of light portable recorders. Ambulation is progressively increased, eventually including longer walks within the hospital premises. The total duration of hospitalization in non-complicated cases is usually between 10 to 14 days. The remainder of the recovery period can be then accomplished at home.

Prior to discharge from the hospital, many physicians perform a low level exercise stress test, during which the patient exercises on the treadmill according to a low level protocol. Although it was once considered dangerous to stress patients soon after an infarction, it has been shown that early stress testing is safe and useful.

The result of the stress test helps the physician to select the proper level of exercise that can be performed safely at home. In addition, the test is often reassuring to patients who may have unrealistic fears about exercising. Finally, by closely watching the patient's symptoms and ECG during this limited stress test, the physician can identify those occasional patients who may be at a higher risk of having recurrence of angina or cardiac arrhythmias during the immediate period following their discharge.

Dissolving the Clot: Streptokinase

The underlying cause of myocardial infarction is atherosclerosis, the progressive build-up of fatty deposits (plaques) inside the coronary arteries. The enlarging plaque itself can lead to critical narrowing of the artery and slowing of blood flow, and may therefore result in severe myocardial ischemia ("starving" of the heart muscle for oxygen). In most cases, however, the immediate cause of infarction is the formation of a fresh blood clot (thrombus) on top of the plaque. This newly formed clot is soft and has the consistency of jello. It "seals off" the coronary artery and thus results in sudden interruption of blood flow to the heart muscle.

When complete interruption of blood flow occurs, the portion of heart muscle supplied by that artery becomes totally deprived of oxygen. If oxygen deprivation is severe or prolonged, it eventually leads to the irreversible damage of the heart muscle. The damage does not happen instantaneously but rather evolves over a period of several hours. Studies have shown that it takes 4 to 6 hours between the formation of a blood clot and the occurrence of irreversible damage to the heart muscle.

Myocardial infarction is a serious condition that can result in major complications, including life-threatening cardiac arrhythmias, "pump failure," and death. It would therefore make sense to try and salvage the ischemic ("starving") heart muscle before the irreversible damage has taken place. This could be accomplished by dissolving the blood clot and re-establishing the blood flow to the heart muscle.

Streptokinase is a powerful drug that has been used to dissolve fresh blood clots. The drug can be introduced directly into the coronary artery (through a catheter) or can be injected into a peripheral vein. When it comes in contact with the clot, it disrupts the microscopic structure of the clot and causes its dissolution. Streptokinase is very effective in dissolving the newly formed blood clot, but it does not eliminate the underlying plaque, on top of which the fresh clot has formed. (See figure 35).

The use of streptokinase is associated with a certain degree of risk (see below). The physician must therefore be reasonably certain of the diagnosis before proceeding with the treatment. The initial diagnosis of a fresh myocardial infarction is based on the presenting symptoms and the ECG findings. The typical candidate has severe and prolonged chest pain, often

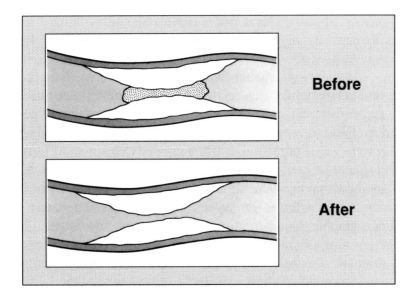

Before

After

Figure 35. Streptokinase is effective in dissolving the newly formed clot, but it does not eliminate the underlying plaque.

associated with sweating, nausea, and shortness of breath. The ECG reveals an "injury pattern" suggestive of an evolving infarction.

In order to be successful, the streptokinase must be given within the first few hours after the onset of symptoms. If given too late, the drug may not be able to salvage the heart muscle tissue from the irreversible damage. In general, the time period during which the drug may be of benefit is about 4 hours. However, the sooner the patient reaches the hospital after the onset of symptoms, the sooner the streptokinase can be given, and the better the chances to salvage the heart muscle. This is another good reason why people with newly developed symptoms of chest pain should seek medical help without delay!

Streptokinase can be injected directly into the coronary artery, through a catheter. After having been examined in the emergency room, the patient is brought to the cardiac catheterization laboratory. A catheter is introduced through the groin (or the arm) and directed toward the opening of the coronary artery. A coronary angiogram is performed, to confirm the presence of a blockage. Streptokinase is then infused directly into the coronary artery, until the blood clot is dissolved. Intracoronary streptoki-nase has a relatively high success rate (around 80 percent). Its major disadvantage is that the preparation for the procedure often delays the treatment. Also, many smaller hospitals do not have the appropriate facilities and personnel for this relatively sophisticated procedure.

An excellent alternative is the injection of streptokinase into a peripheral vein, through the intravenous line. This can be done in the emergency room or in the coronary care unit (CCU). The major advantage of the intravenous approach is that treatment can be initiated within minutes after the diagnosis is made, therefore saving valuable time. The relative disadvantages of this approach are a somewhat lower success rate (around 70 percent), and the lack of angiographic documentation of the coronary blockage.

The re-opening of the coronary artery (reperfusion) with streptokinase is often dramatic. Within minutes after successful reperfusion, there is usually a sudden relief of chest pain and a rapid return of the ECG toward normal. Some patients may develop serious cardiac arrhythmias, but these are generally transient, and can be treated with drugs.

The major risk from streptokinase is bleeding. This powerful substance interferes with the person's own clotting mechanism, and will therefore prevent the clotting of blood that normally occurs after injury or surgery. In order to minimize the risk, streptokinase is generally contraindicated in patients with a recent history of active internal bleeding or major surgery.

Second generation clot-dissolving drugs, which appear to be more effective than streptokinase, are now being extensively tested. The greatest attention has focused on TPA (tissue-type plasminogen activator), which is more selective than streptokinase in dissolving blood clots, and therefore causes fewer allergic reactions and a lesser risk of serious bleeding.

As mentioned above, streptokinase is effective in dissolving the newly formed clot, but it does not eliminate the underlying plaque (see figure 35). Following successful reperfusion, there remains a significant narrowing of the coronary artery, and therefore a constant threat of a new infarction. In a way, streptokinase is just a palliative procedure that allows to "buy time." For this reason, a coronary angiogram is generally performed in the days following a successful streptokinase treatment. If significant coronary artery disease is found, then the patient may be a candidate for additional procedures, such as coronary balloon angioplasty or bypass surgery.

Complications of the M.I.

Two general types of complications can occur in the setting of a myocardial infarction :

a) Electrical complications, caused by disruption of the electrical system in the heart.

b) Mechanical complications, resulting from the damage to the ventricular heart muscle.

Electrical complications

Most patients admitted to the hospital with an acute ("fresh") myocardial infarction will have some type of cardiac arrhythmia, especially during the first 24 hours. The heart may beat too slowly (bradycardia), or too rapidly (tachycardia), or it may become erratic. Some cardiac arrhythmias are benign and of no major consequence, but other arrhythmias can be extremely serious and may lead to death if not treated promptly. (For more information on cardiac arrhythmias, see Chapter 17).

During myocardial infarction, portions of the injured heart muscle in the ventricle may become irritable and may discharge or "fire" independently. When the irritable site fires, the result is a beat that occurs before the next expected normal beat. This "extra beat" is termed a *premature ventricular contraction* (or *PVC*). Extra beats are generally of no major consequence, and are often seen in healthy individuals. In the setting of a myocardial infarction, however, PVCs can be dangerous. In fact, if not treated promptly, they can lead to more serious arrhythmias, such as ventricular tachycardia and ventricular fibrillation (see below). If treatment is required, these PVCs can be suppressed effectively with drugs (such as Lidocaine) injected directly into the vein.

If the irritable site in the ventricle discharges repetitively at a fast rate, it may lead to a potentially more serious arrhythmia, called *ventricular tachycardia*. If the rapid heart beat persists, the volume of blood pumped by the ventricle may decrease dangerously, and unless successfully controlled, this may lead to rapid deterioration of the patient's condition. Ventricular tachycardia can be terminated with Lidocaine injected into the vein. If the tachycardia persists, or if there is evidence of deterioration of the patient's condition, electrical cardioversion (an electric shock delivered through the chest wall) is indicated without delay.

When a group of irritable sites in the ventricle start firing very rapidly and erratically, the result is a life-threatening arrhythmia, called *ventricular fibrillation*. The ventricles are unable to respond completely and effectively to each stimulus, and as a result there is a very rapid, irregular, uncoordinated twitching of the heart muscle. Ventricular fibrillation is equivalent to cardiac arrest: there is no pulse or breathing, and the patient loses consciousness. If normal rhythm is not restored immediately, death follows within a few minutes. Emergency electrical shock (defibrillation) is the only effective treatment for ventricular fibrillation, and it must be performed promptly, otherwise the chances for survival are very small.

Another type of arrhythmia commonly seen in the setting of a heart attack is *bradycardia*, that is, an excessively slow heartbeat. Bradycardia can occur either as a result of inordinate slowing of the heart's natural pacemaker (sinus bradycardia) or from disruption of the heart's conduction system (heart block). The slow heart rate leads to inadequate delivery of blood to the brain, heart muscle, and other vital organs. Bradycardia can be treated with drugs (such as atropine) injected through the vein. When bradycardia is severe, however, or when it is the result of a heart block, atropine may not be effective, and the insertion of a temporary pacemaker may be necessary. The pacemaker is a device consisting of a battery that produces the electrical impulses, and a wire that transmits these impulses to the ventricle to stimulate it when slowing down (see Chapter 17).

Mechanical Complications

Myocardial infarction results in irreversible damage to an area of the heart muscle and loss of a functioning segment of the ventricular wall. When the damage is significant, it may result in symptoms of *congestive heart failure:* the heart muscle is unable to pump a sufficient amount of blood to maintain adequate circulation. The weakened ventricle does not empty properly, and blood returning to it backs up and collects in the lungs, thus leading to congestion of the lungs. Heart failure can generally be controlled with various cardiovascular drugs. Diuretic medications, for example, enhance the urine flow and result in improvement of the congestion. Cardiac stimulant drugs are used to improve the force of contraction of the heart muscle. Vasodilator drugs reduce the workload on the heart and can therefore improve cardiac performance.

When the damage to the heart muscle is extensive, this often leads to the collapse of the entire circulatory system, a condition known as *cardiogenic shock* (or "pump failure"). This is an extreme form of heart failure, in which the weakened heart is unable to pump a sufficient amount of blood to maintain an adequate blood pressure. Cardiogenic shock is a very serious condition, which carries an extremely poor outlook. Even with "aggressive" medical therapy, the death rate is over 80 percent. The treatment of cardiogenic shock is complex, and it usually requires the expertise of a well trained cardiologist.

The damage to the heart muscle from the fresh infarction can occasionally lead to breaking (rupture) of the heart muscle, a condition termed *myocardial rupture*. When the rupture involves the free wall of the left ventricle, the consequence is usually immediate death. When the rupture involves an area of the septum (the muscular wall between the two ventricles) or a portion of the mitral valve apparatus, it usually leads to severe leakage of blood and inefficient pumping of the ventricles. These complications are extremely serious and often lead to progressive heart failure, cardiogenic shock, and death. In some patients, the leakage can be repaired with cardiac surgery. This type of surgical procedure, however, is technically difficult and is often associated with an extremely high risk.

Other Complications

In some patients with a recent heart attack, the damaged heart muscle tissue becomes weakened and thin and may begin to "balloon out," creating a sac-like area in the wall of the ventricle, termed a *ventricular aneurysm*. This portion of the heart muscle does not contract properly and bulges out with each contraction of the ventricle, thus decreasing the efficiency of the heart pump. Ventricular aneurysms are generally well tolerated. In some patients, however, their presence may lead to chronic manifestations of heart failure and recurrent cardiac arrhythmias.

A potentially serious complication in patients with a fresh myocardial infarction is the *formation of blood clots* within the heart chambers. When the damage to the heart muscle is significant, a portion of the ventricular wall becomes "sluggish" or immobile. The blood flow near the damaged area is slowed down, and this may lead to the formation of blood clots attached to the inside of the wall. If these blood clots become dislodged, they may travel through the bloodstream and may eventually cause damage to distant organs (such as the brain, kidneys, intestines, and extremities). When the presence of blood clots within the heart is confirmed or strongly suspected, treatment is started with "blood thinners" (anticoagulant drugs). These drugs delay the clotting of blood and prevent the formation of additional blood clots.

A relatively common complication seen in patients with fresh myocardial infarction is the inflammation of the thin membrane that surrounds the heart (pericardium), a condition called *pericarditis*. (See also Chapter 21). Pericarditis, when it happens, usually occurs a few days after the infarction, and is manifested by the onset of recurrent chest pain. The pain of pericarditis is typically worsened by deep breathing and by turning in bed. Pericarditis in the setting of a heart attack is generally a temporary condition, which usually responds to treatment with anti-inflammatory drugs (such as aspirin).

Recovery: After a Heart Attack

After a heart attack, the body sets out to repair the damaged heart muscle. The healing process, during which scar tissue replaces the infarcted heart muscle, requires about six to eight weeks. The recovery period allows patients to regain their strength and stamina. It takes about two to three months for most patients to get back to "normal" following a heart attack. However, the severity of the infarction, the rate of healing, and the general strength and stamina vary from patient to patient. Consequently, the time it takes to recover will also vary. (For further information on recovery after a heart attack, see Chapter 25).

15 High Blood Pressure

High blood pressure, also known as hypertension, is a condition characterized by an excessive amount of pressure within the arteries. It is one of the most common medical problems in this country, affecting 15 to 20 percent of the adult population. In most patients, the elevated blood pressure produces no symptoms (it is "silent"). If not treated, however, it can lead to progressive damage to the blood vessels and to other vital organs (especially the heart, brain, and kidneys). In fact, it is estimated that hypertensive people are five times more likely to have a heart attack than people whose blood pressure is normal. For these reasons, hypertension has often been referred to as the "silent killer."

Blood pressure is the force of blood against the walls of the arteries, created by the heart as it pumps blood to all parts of the body. The walls of the arteries are elastic, so they stretch then contract to take the ups and downs of the blood pressure. When the blood pressure is measured, two pressures are recorded in numbers (such as "120 over 80"). The higher number, called the systolic pressure, is generated when the left ventricle (the main pumping chamber) contracts and ejects blood under pressure into the arterial system. The lower number, termed the diastolic pressure, is produced when the left ventricle relaxes between two beats, as the pressure within the arteries gradually falls.

There is a wide variation of blood pressure levels among individuals. In a given person there is, in addition, a variation of blood pressure throughout the day. During physical activity and emotional stress, for example, the blood pressure tends to rise. During resting periods and sleep, on the other hand, it tends to be lower.

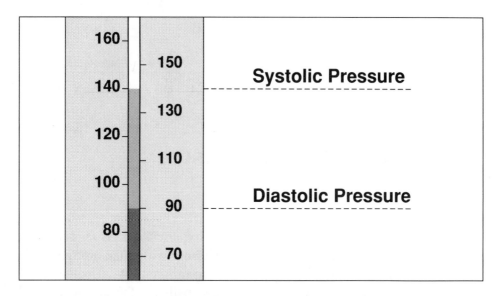

Figure 36. Blood pressure readings of 140/90 are generally considered to be at the upper limit of normal.

While there is no clear definition of where "normal" ends, and where "abnormal" begins, most physicians use readings of 140/90 as the upper limit of normal (see figure 36). Blood pressure readings between 140/90 and 160/95 are generally considered "borderline." The diagnosis of hypertension should not be based on an isolated reading, but should be substantiated by repeated readings, on separate occasions.

The Causes of Hypertension

In the most common form of hypertension, a specific cause cannot be found, and the condition is termed "essential" (or primary) hypertension. Although the cause is unknown, several factors have been implicated in the development of hypertension, including heredity, salt intake, obesity, and stress. In a small number of patients with hypertension, a specific cause can be identified, and the condition is then termed "secondary" hypertension. Nearly all the secondary forms are related to either an alteration in kidney function or an excessive secretion of certain hormones.

Essential Hypertension

Essential hypertension is by far the most common cause of high blood pressure, being present in over 90 percent of cases. Although the specific cause of essential hypertension is not known, the mechanisms involved have been well defined.

In general terms, the blood pressure is determined by the relation between the amount of blood pumped by the heart (cardiac output), and the resistance of the peripheral arteries to blood flow (peripheral resistance). An elevation of the blood pressure may occur either from an increase in the amount of blood pumped by the heart, or from the constriction (tightening) of the peripheral arteries.

The blood pressure is controlled and regulated by a complex control system. The heart, kidneys, and autonomic (or involuntary) nervous system all play an important part in regulating the blood pressure. The control system acts to keep the pressure within a certain "preset" range: it senses when the pressure is too low or too high and makes whatever adjustments are necessary by releasing certain chemical substances (hormones), or by stimulating the autonomic nervous system.

Various disturbances in body functions can affect the cardiac output and the peripheral resistance, and may thus cause hypertension. The nature of these disturbances varies widely among individuals, but generally include one or more of the following: increased contractility (force of contraction) of the heart; excessive amount of salt and fluid within the body; increased levels of certain hormones; and excessive stimulation of the autonomic nervous system. The interaction between these various mechanisms is extremely complex, and it is often difficult to separate cause and effect.

Several factors have been implicated in the development and progression of hypertension, including:

Heredity. It appears that a tendency to develop high blood pressure is passed from parent to child. A person who had one or two hypertensive parents, for example, does have a higher chance of developing high blood pressure, compared to a person who did not have hypertensive parents.

Salt intake. People living in modern industrialized countries tend to consume an excessive amount of salt (often 10 to 20 times the amount needed by the body!). In studies of large populations, the prevalence of hypertension tends to increase with higher levels of salt intake. It is therefore likely that high salt intake is responsible, at least to some degree, for many cases of hypertension. Salt restriction will lower the blood pressure in most hypertensive patients, and is often used in the management of mild hypertension.

Obesity. High blood pressure is more common among obese individuals. Obese children and adults have an increased likelihood of developing hypertension compared to people of normal weight. Weight loss in obese individuals is often helpful in controlling an elevated blood pressure level.

Stress. In some individuals, a high level of emotional stress may worsen their hypertension. The relief of stress by relaxation techniques has been shown to reduce blood pressure, at least temporarily, in many hypertensive persons. Decreased exposure to stress or improved ways of dealing with stress may therefore help lower the blood pressure in those individuals.

Secondary Hypertension

A specific cause for hypertension can be found in only a small minority (less than 10 percent) of patients with elevated blood pressure. It is important to identify that cause, since its correction will result in the cure of the hypertensive state. Nearly all the secondary forms of hypertension are related to either an alteration in kidney function or to an excessive secretion of adrenal hormones.

The kidneys are vital organs whose main function is to remove waste products from the bloodstream. The kidneys also take part in the control of salt and water metabolism. By constantly changing the composition of the urine, the kidneys are able to regulate the composition of the fluids within the blood and body tissues. When there exists an excess of salt and/or water in the body, for example, the kidneys increase the filtration of salt and/or water into the urine, thus correcting the body's fluid balance.

The kidneys are also involved in the regulation of the blood pressure through a complex mechanism (the renin-angiotensin system). The kidneys secrete a hormone-like substance, called renin, that has an important role in the regulation of blood pressure. Following its release into the circulation, renin acts on a circulating protein to produce angiotensin, a naturally occurring substance that induces an elevation of the blood pressure through two different mechanisms: tightening (constriction) of the peripheral blood vessels, and retention of salt and water.

Several forms of secondary hypertension are due to the presence of excessive amounts of certain hormones in the body. A hormone is a substance produced within the body and carried by the blood to the organ which it stimulates. The adrenal glands (located just above the kidneys) normally secrete several hormones (such as cortisol, adrenalin, and aldosterone) which play an important role in the control of the blood pressure level. An excessive production of these adrenal hormones can lead to a rise in the blood pressure level.

As already mentioned, most secondary forms of hypertension are due to either an alteration in kidney function or an excessive amount of certain hormones within the body. The most frequent causes of secondary hypertension are:

• *Chronic kidney disease.* Damage to the kidneys often results in elevation of the blood pressure. Hypertension produced by kidney disease is generally the result of a disturbance in the handling of salt and water by the damaged kidneys, leading to an excessive amount of fluids in the body. Other times, it is due to an excessive secretion of substances (similar to renin) that induce constriction of the peripheral arteries, and thus elevate the blood pressure.

• *Renovascular hypertension.* There is an abnormal narrowing of one or both renal arteries, most commonly due to atherosclerosis. The resulting decrease in blood flow to the corresponding kidney(s) leads to stimulation of renin production, and thus to elevation of the blood pressure.

• *Overproduction of hormones by the adrenal glands.* Various diseases of the adrenal glands can lead to excessive production of one or more adrenal hormones (cortisol, adrenalin, or aldosterone). Each one of these hormones may result in changes of bodily functions leading to the elevation of the blood pressure.

• *Use of oral contraceptives.* The prolonged use of the "pill" can occasionally result in elevation of the blood pressure. However, only a small percentage of the women using birth control pills will ever develop significant hypertension.

The Effects of Hypertension

Long-standing elevation of the blood pressure in hypertensive patients may lead to an acceleration of the atherosclerotic process, that is, the deposit of plaques in the walls of the arteries. This process is especially common in the aorta (the body's main artery) and in the major arterial branches conducting blood to vital organs, such as the heart, brain, and kidneys. It is therefore not surprising that hypertensive patients have a significantly higher risk of developing heart attacks, strokes, and kidney disease.

Chronic elevation of the blood pressure also leads to progressive structural changes in the small peripheral arteries (arterioles). These changes may include an increased thickness of the arteriolar wall and a narrowing of the channel. The result is an increased resistance to blood flow, and therefore an extra strain on the heart.

Long-standing hypertension, especially if untreated, eventually results in damage to one or more vital organs, termed "target organs:"

Effects on the Heart. As we have seen, high blood pressure is a major risk factor in the development of coronary heart disease, that is, the build-up of atherosclerotic plaques within the coronary arteries (see Chapter 2). Total blockage of a coronary artery may in turn result in damage to an area of the heart muscle (myocardial infarction or heart attack).

The heart may also suffer from the constant strain of having to pump blood against higher resistance. Over the years, this pressure burden leads to thickening (hypertrophy) of the ventricular wall, thereby strengthening the force of its contraction. If left untreated, however, hypertension may lead to the development of congestive heart failure, a condition in which the heart is unable to pump sufficient blood to maintain adequate delivery of oxygen and nutrients to the body.

Effects on the Brain. Hypertension is a major risk factor for the development of strokes. A stroke results from the total obstruction of blood flow in one of the arteries conducting blood to the brain. Other times, it may result from the rupture (bursting) of a blood vessel, followed by a hemorrhage (bleeding) into the brain tissue. In either case, the damaged brain tissue cannot function properly, and manifestations of a stroke (such as weakness of a limb, paralysis, or loss of speech) develop.

Effects on the Kidneys. Being rich in blood vessels, the kidneys are particularly susceptible to the damaging effects of hypertension. The long-standing elevation of the blood pressure leads to a progressive narrowing of the small arteries (arterioles) within the kidneys. As a result, the kidneys are unable to function properly, and waste products accumulate in the bloodstream, eventually leading to kidney failure.

Effects on the Eyes. The layered lining of the eye (retina), containing the light-sensitive receptors, is rich in tiny blood vessels (arterioles). Long-standing hypertension can cause serious eye problems, such as bleeding (retinal hemorrages) or the formation of blood clots in the tiny blood vessels. Depending on the exact location of the problem in the eye, these complications can cause no symptoms or they can cause reduced vision and blindness. The changes in the retina often mirror more serious changes elsewhere in the body, especially in the heart, brain, and kidneys.

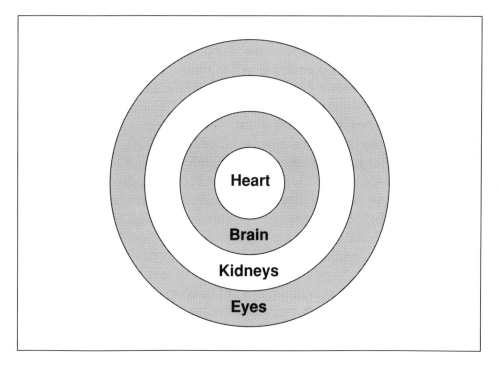

Figure 37. Long-standing hypertension may result in damage to one or more vital organs, termed "target organs."

Clinical Evaluation of Hypertension

The majority of patients with hypertension have no symptoms referable to their high blood pressure! In fact, hypertension is generally diagnosed when the blood pressure is measured in the course of a routine physical examination. When symptoms do occur, they are often variable and nonspecific. Some patients, for example, may develop recurrent headaches (typically upon awakening in the morning), may become fatigued easily, or may complain of dizziness, blurring of vision, or nose bleeds.

The clinical evaluation of patients with hypertension has three major objectives:

- Establish the presence of hypertension
- Determine the amount of damage to "target organs"
- Uncover correctable (secondary) forms of hypertension

Establishing the Presence of Hypertension

The most important step in the diagnosis of hypertension is the *measurement of the blood pressure.* (See figure 38). To take a pressure reading, the doctor uses a blood pressure machine (sphygmomanometer), and a stethoscope. The sphygmomanometer has two main parts: a rubber cuff which encircles the patient's arm, and a gauge that measures the pressure within the cuff. (See also pages 172 and 173).

As the pressure is slowly released by opening a valve, the pressure in the cuff gradually falls. When the pressure within the cuff falls just below the upper level of the blood pressure (the systolic pressure), a spurt of blood escapes from the compressed artery with each heartbeat, producing a thumping sound heard through the stethoscope. The level of blood pressure when the thumping sound begins is the systolic pressure, which can be read as a result of its effect against either a column of mercury or an air gauge. The pressure is expressed in millimeters of mercury (mmHg), which is how high the column of mercury is pushed by the pressure of the blood. A normal systolic pressure is around 120 mmHg.

As more of the air in the blood pressure cuff is released, more and more blood squirts through the artery into the forearm, continuing to produce a thumping sound with each heartbeat. When the pressure in the cuff falls

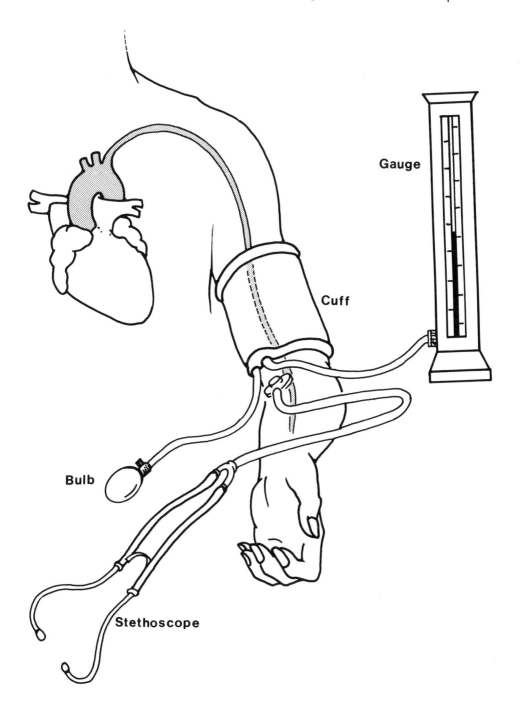

Figure 38. The measurement of blood pressure.

below the lower level of the blood pressure (the diastolic pressure), there is no further obstruction to blood flow, and the thumping sound disappears. The level of blood pressure when the sound disappears is the diastolic pressure. A normal diastolic pressure is around 80 mmHg.

The result, in this example, is a normal blood pressure of 120/80 mmHg, expressed as "one-twenty over eighty." It should be emphasized that one's blood pressure varies during the course of the day, and readings taken just minutes apart may be 10 to 20 mmHg different from one another. Some of these differences may be due to excitement, nervousness, or physical activity. The blood pressure levels also vary according to the time of day. During sleep, for example, blood pressure tends to be lower than during the time a person is awake.

Before a definitive diagnosis of hypertension can be made, the physician should obtain multiple readings, on separate occasions. However, even an occasional high reading shouldn't be ignored, because it may be a warning signal that more persistent hypertension is developing.

As part of a *complete physical examination,* the physician will carefully examine the cardiovascular system. During the examination of the heart and lungs, he will search for evidence of cardiac enlargement or signs of heart failure. In patients with heart failure, the lungs become congested, and crackling sounds (rales) can be heard during breathing when a stethoscope is applied over the chest. A systematic examination of the arterial pulses in the neck and extremities is also important. A weak or absent pulse may represent a narrowing or blockage of that artery by a plaque.

The *examination of the "eye grounds"* (fundi) with a bright light will provide important information about the condition of the tiny arteries (arterioles) inside the eyes. Normally, these arterioles appear red, as a result of the column of blood they contain. In cases of long-standing hypertension, these vessels undergo typical changes, including the thickening of the arteriolar wall, giving the appearance of "copper wires." Severe and progressive hypertension may also induce rupture of these small vessels, seen as small areas of bleeding (hemorrhage) in the eye ground.

Diagnostic Tests in Patients with Hypertension

Several basic tests are performed routinely in all patients with hypertension. In selected patients, when the initial evaluation is suggestive of a secondary form of hypertension, more specialized studies will be done.

The *basic studies* include several laboratory tests that are useful in assessing the function of the vital organs, especially the kidneys and the heart. The kidney function can be assessed by obtaining several blood tests (such as serum creatinine and blood urea nitrogen), and by examining the urine for the abnormal presence of protein, sugar, blood, and cells. The two basic tests used to evaluate the cardiac function are the electrocardiogram (ECG) and the chest x-ray. In patients with long-standing hypertension, the ECG may show evidence of ventricular hypertrophy (thickening of the ventricular walls). In these patients, the chest x-ray may reveal an enlargement of the heart shadow.

When the initial clinical evaluation (history, physical examination, and basic laboratory studies) suggests the presence of a secondary form of hypertension, *specialized studies* may be indicated. When renovascular hypertension is suspected, for example, the physician may order specialized x-rays of the kidneys (intravenous pyelogram, or IVP). If the IVP is abnormal, a more definite diagnosis can be obtained by performing more sophisticated tests, such as a renal angiogram (the injection of dye and visualization of the renal arteries).

When overproduction of hormones (such as cortisol, adrenalin, or aldosterone) by the adrenal glands is suspected, the physician may order specialized studies to measure the level of these hormones in the blood.

As already mentioned above, the secondary forms of hypertension are found in less than 10 percent of hypertensive patients. Therefore, these specialized (and usually expensive) tests are generally reserved for patients whose initial evaluation suggests a secondary form of hypertension.

Treatment of Hypertension

The main reason for treating hypertension is to prevent its potential consequences. Even in its mild form, hypertension is a progressive disease that leads to a significant increase in the risk of developing cardiovascular complications. Studies have shown that long-standing untreated hypertension is associated with a shortening of life by 10 years or more. It has been shown that patients with severe hypertension may have a significant reduction in disability and mortality if started on a treatment program.

There is no clear-cut dividing line between "normal" and "abnormal" levels of blood pressure. Generally, the higher the pressure, the higher the risk of developing cardiovascular complications. Arbitrary levels of blood pressure have been established in order to define those patients who may have an increased risk of developing complications and may thus benefit from medical treatment.

It has been shown that the use of the diastolic pressure (the "low number") is more reliable than the systolic pressure (the "high number") in terms of correlating between the blood pressure level and the risk of cardiovascular complications. In general, most physicians will recommend treatment in patients with a diastolic pressure repeatedly above 95 and/or a systolic pressure above 160 mmHg.

In patients with a diastolic pressure between 90 and 95 and/or a systolic pressure between 140 and 160 mmHg, the decision whether or not to treat is more difficult, and depends on each individual case. In this "borderline" group, treatment is usually recommended in persons who are relatively young, in those who have already suffered some target organ damage, and in those who have additional risk factors for cardiovascular disease (such as elevated cholesterol level, cigarette smoking, or obesity).

Some doctors have their patients measure their own blood pressure at home. This may be especially helpful during the early stages, when the doctor has to know how much the pressure varies during the day or how the body reacts to certain blood pressure medications. Some patients will be encouraged to continue the monitoring of their blood pressure after a treatment program has been established.

The equipment needed for home blood pressure measurement consists of two components: 1) a sphygmomanometer, a device which measures the pressure in the artery, and 2) a stethoscope, which detects the sound of blood as it moves through the artery. Most digital readout devices have the stethoscope built into the cuff.

The sphygmomanometer includes four basic parts: a) a cuff, which encircles the arm and encloses an inflatable rubber bag; b) a gauge (either mercury column, air gauge, or digital readout) that indicates the pressure applied and the reading obtained; c) an inflation bulb, that allows air to be pumped into the cuff; and d) a control valve, which adjusts the rate of deflation of the cuff.

How to Measure Your Own Blood Pressure

• Pick a quiet spot. Sit comfortably next to a table, and rest your forearm flat on the table.

• Use your fingers to locate the artery at the bend of the elbow. Feel for the pulse, a little to the inside of the center of the elbow's crease. This is the best place for the stethoscope.

• Slip on the deflated cuff, placing the stethoscope over the artery. Use the ring or velcro wrap to make the cuff snug. Place the stethoscope in your ears. You can test it by gently tapping the stethoscope with your finger and finding the best position for the ear pieces.

• You are now ready to inflate the cuff, by squeezing the rubber bulb rapidly. Inflate the cuff roughly 30 "points" (millimeters of mercury) above the expected systolic pressure. This value will be determined by trial and error. Since most people know about where their pressure is, it is easy for them to decide how high to inflate the cuff.

• Once the cuff pressure is greater than your systolic pressure, you will not hear any sound in the stethoscope. In effect, you have made a tourniquet for your arm and have cut off all of the blood supply.

• Keeping your eyes on the gauge, slowly release the pressure in the cuff, using the release knob on the bulb.

• As the cuff pressure falls, it will continue to act as a tourniquet as long as its pressure is greater than the arterial pressure. When the cuff pressure drops below the arterial pressure, a pulse beat gets through, and you will hear the sound of that pulse. Read the gauge level at the time you hear the first sound. This is the systolic pressure.

• Continue to let air out. The thumping sound, corresponding to the pulse wave that gets through the tourniquet, will first get louder as more blood gets by. Then, as the cuff pressure approaches diastolic pressure, the sound gets faint until it disappears. The gauge reading at the time of the last sound is the diastolic pressure.

• You may take a second reading after a one-minute wait. Record date, time, systolic and diastolic pressures.

General Measures

The following measures are indicated in all patients with hypertension, whether or not they are candidates for drug treatment. For some patients with borderline hypertension, these measures will be sufficient to bring the blood pressure down to a safe level. In others, these steps may be only partially effective, but will surely benefit the general physical health of the patient. Since these measures often require a change in lifestyle, they should be introduced gradually and gently. Too many or too drastic changes in lifestyle may discourage patients from accepting much needed care.

As we saw, it is very likely that high salt intake is responsible, at least in part, for many cases of hypertension. *Restriction of salt intake* is therefore advisable in most hypertensive patients. The desired degree of salt restriction can be easily accomplished by most patients by having them follow several simple guidelines: not adding salt to food during cooking or at the table; avoiding obviously salty foods such as pickles, sauerkraut, and salted peanuts; avoiding or minimizing the use of canned or prepacked foods, to which an undue amount of salt has been added; and recognizing the salt (sodium) content of various foods, antacids, and drugs, by reading the package labels.

In obese individuals, *weight loss* is an effective way of reducing the blood pressure. In general, the degree of reduction in blood pressure correlates with the degree of weight loss. The discovery that they have hypertension may be a strong motivation for obese persons to lose weight. In most patients, the biggest problem with weight control is not necessarily how to lose a few pounds, but rather how to keep those extra pounds off for extended periods of time. Therefore, a weight reduction program should stress the importance of changing the patient's underlying eating habits, by a carefully thought-out behavior modification program.

Besides promoting a general sense of well-being, *regular exercise* may help lower the blood pressure by burning up excess calories and helping in weight loss. The recommended type of exercise is the "aerobic" type, such as walking, jogging, and swimming. During aerobic exercise, the systolic blood pressure usually goes up but the diastolic pressure stays at the same level or may go down. To obtain a full conditioning effect, a moderate level of exercise should last for at least 20 to 30 minutes, and should be repeated several times a week. An isometric type of exercise, such as weight-lifting, may be harmful to hypertensive patients, since it often results in significant (although temporary) elevation of the blood pressure.

The relief of stress by way of *relaxation* may reduce the blood pressure, at least temporarily, in many hypertensive persons. Relaxation can be achieved by reducing exposure to stress; for example, by working fewer hours or taking more vacation time. Various types of relaxation techniques (such as meditation and biofeedback) have been used with some success to improve the ways of dealing with stress. Hypertensive patients should be encouraged to *quit smoking*. Although cigarette smoking has little direct effect on the blood pressure itself, it is another major risk factor for the development of cardiovascular disease.

Drug Therapy

The goal of therapy is to reduce the blood pressure to normal (that is, below 140/90 mmHg) without inducing troublesome side effects. The physician's decision whether or not to use drugs is generally based on several factors, such as the level of the blood pressure, the patient's age, the presence of target organ damage, and the presence of other cardiovascular risk factors. In patients with mild hypertension, the short-term risk from cardiovascular complications is small, and the use of non-drug treatment is generally adequate. On the other hand, when the diastolic pressure is consistently above 100 mmHg, particularly when it is accompanied by target organ damage or other major risk factors, drug treatment is indicated without delay.

The drugs used in the treatment of hypertension are quite effective, and will reduce the blood pressure level in most hypertensive patients. Because of their potency, however, these drugs can cause bothersome side effects and adverse reactions. Although antihypertensive drugs will lower the blood pressure in most patients, they do not "cure" the disease. Because of the chronic nature of hypertension and its slow progression into a heart attack or stroke, drug treatment will almost certainly be lifelong. Patients are therefore advised not to stop taking their medication just because they have been feeling well.

Five major classes of drugs, each with a different mechanism of action, are currently used in the treatment of hypertension: diuretics, beta blockers, centrally-acting drugs, vasodilators, and angiotensin inhibitors. The "stepped-care approach" (see below), beginning with the mildest treatment and then proceeding to increasingly more potent drugs until adequate control is achieved, is the most effective way of treating hypertension.

Diuretics. The diuretics ("water pills") act primarily by increasing the elimination of salt and water into the urine, leading to reduction of the amount of fluid in the circulation, and thus a lowering of the blood pressure. Many physicians use a diuretic as the first-step drug in the initial treatment of mild hypertension. A diuretic is often added to other antihypertensive drugs when a combination of several medications is needed to control the blood pressure. The major side effect resulting from the use of diuretics is the undesired loss ("wasting") of potassium in the urine, which may lead to symptoms of leg cramps, fatigue, and palpitations. If loss of potassium is a problem, potassium supplements are generally prescribed together with the diuretic agent.

Beta Blockers. Beta blockers are rapidly becoming the most popular form of antihypertensive therapy. These agents act predominantly by blocking the stimulation of the beta receptors (the nerve endings that affect the heart rate and the force of cardiac contraction), thus leading to decreased cardiac output and lowering of the blood pressure. In addition, they act at the level of the central nervous system, reducing the outflow of stimulation to the peripheral arteries, causing them to dilate. A beta blocker can be either prescribed as a first-step drug in the initial treatment of hypertension, or it can be added as a second drug in patients who were previously treated with a diuretic alone. Common side effects of the beta blockers include fatigue, shortness of breath, wheezing, and dizziness.

Centrally-Acting Drugs. These are substances that lower the blood pressure by blocking the transmission of impulses within the autonomic nervous system (which controls the involuntary action of various internal organs, including the heart, lungs, and blood vessels). Because of their potency, these drugs have a higher incidence of side effects. They are usually reserved for patients with more severe forms of hypertension who have not responded to treatment with milder medications. The most troublesome side effect encountered in this group is postural hypotension, that is, a sudden drop of blood pressure upon standing up, which may lead to bothersome symptoms of lightheadedness and faintness.

Vasodilators. They lower blood pressure by relaxing the vascular smooth muscle of the peripheral arteries, thus causing them to dilate. As a result of vascular dilatation, the resistance to blood flow is reduced, and the blood pressure is lowered. These potent drugs are generally prescribed to patients with severe hypertension, and are usually given in combination with other agents, such as beta blockers and diuretics. The major drawback of vasodilator drugs is their tendency to cause a reflex acceleration of the heart rate, as well as retention of salt and water. The addition of a beta blocker helps prevent the reflex increase in heart rate, and the addition of a diuretic is used to overcome the tendency for salt and water retention.

Angiotensin Inhibitors. These drugs lower blood pressure through inhibition of the renin-angiotensin system. As we have seen, renin is a hormone-like substance that is normally secreted by the kidneys. Following its release into the circulation, renin acts on a circulating protein to produce angiotensin, a naturally occurring substance that induces an elevation of the blood pressure through two different mechanisms: tightening (constriction) of the peripheral blood vessels, and retention of salt and water.

The angiotensin-inhibitor drugs lower the blood pressure by blocking the actions of angiotensin. The use of these agents is associated with a relatively high incidence of adverse reactions, especially hypotension (low blood pressure), skin rashes, and kidney problems. Their use is therefore reserved for patients with the more severe forms of hypertension, when other agents have not been effective in lowering the blood pressure.

. . . .

The *"stepped-care approach"* in the treatment of hypertension refers to the addition of drugs, stepwise, in sufficient doses to achieve the goals of therapy. Most physicians use either a diuretic or a beta blocker as a first-step drug in the initial treatment of hypertension. Then, if the blood pressure is not adequately controlled with either drug alone, a second drug is added. The combination of a diuretic and a beta blocker, for example, is quite effective, lowering the blood pressure in the great majority of hypertensive patients. The other antihypertensive agents (centrally-acting drugs, vasodilators, and angiotensin inhibitors) are usually reserved for hypertensive patients who have not tolerated or have not responded to treatment with a diuretic or a beta blocker (or a combination of the two).

Guidelines: Controlling Your High Blood Pressure

• Whether or not you are asked to take medications to lower your blood pressure, the effective use of non-drug treatment is of utmost importance. Cut down on salt! Lose weight! Exercise regularly! Give up smoking! Learn to relax!

• Hypertension is a chronic disease. Therefore, treatment will almost certainly be lifelong. Keep taking your medications even if you feel perfectly well, particularly if you feel perfectly well!

• Have your blood pressure checked every few weeks, even after you have achieved good control. Don't be concerned if the pressure fluctuates somewhat between visits; it may reflect nothing more than temporary stress or a normal variation.

• The use of antihypertensive drugs is commonly associated with side effects. They are generally mild and temporary. If you feel you are experiencing a side effect, don't just stop treatment. Call your doctor and discuss the matter with him.

• Take your medications as directed. Try taking them routinely at the same time of the day, so you won't forget. It is so easy to forget, particularly when you feel well.

• If you and your doctor have agreed that you should take your blood pressure at home, follow the directions. Remember, however, that home blood pressure measurement is not a substitute for periodic evaluation by your doctor or other medical professionals.

• Don't change your medications on the basis of changes in your home readings without first checking with your doctor.

• If you happened to miss a dose or two, don't take all the doses you have missed at one time to make up for the loss. Just get back on the prescribed schedule.

• It may take some time and effort to achieve the treatment goals. The reward for your efforts is the knowledge that effective control of hypertension will eventually lead to a healthier and longer life.

After blood pressure has been lowered and is under control, a few changes may be made that can make the medication schedule more convenient. Many drugs for high blood pressure are combined in fixed dosages into a single tablet or capsule, providing the advantage of ingesting a smaller number of pills. These so-called "combination drugs" are usually prescribed only after the individual ingredients have been tried successfully first. Most of these combination drugs combine a diuretic with another antihypertensive drug.

A serious problem in treating hypertension is that many people simply stop taking medications that have been prescribed. Some patients may have trouble accepting the fact that they indeed have a medical problem when they have no symptoms. Others stop their treatment without discussing the problem with their doctor, after having experienced bothersome side effects. Other times, blood pressure is successfully lowered with treatment, and the patients mistakenly think that they are "cured" and no longer need the medication. Patients who stop taking their medications offer a variety of excuses, including statements such as "schedules are not convenient;" "medications are too expensive;" "I forgot to take the medicine;" and "I'm afraid of becoming dependent on the drug."

The short-term goal of treatment is to lower the blood pressure and to keep it under control. In the vast majority of people with hypertension, the blood pressure can be controlled with a simple combination of drugs and with a minimum number of side effects. The ultimate objective of treatment, however, is the prevention of potential cardiovascular complications (such as heart attacks and strokes) resulting from untreated hypertension. This objective is best achieved when patients accept the fact that they have hypertension, when they understand what hypertension is, and when they decide that their health is important and that the benefits of treatment eventually outweigh the difficulties.

16 Congestive Heart Failure

Congestive heart failure is a condition in which the weakened heart is unable to pump sufficient blood to maintain adequate delivery of oxygen and nutrients to the body tissues. The term "failure" does not necessarily imply imminent death from heart disease! It simply means that the pumping function of the heart is impaired. When the heart cannot pump enough blood, there is a backup of blood in the lungs, resulting in congestion of the lungs and other tissues.

Causes of Heart Failure

It is useful to separate the causes of congestive heart failure into two separate categories:

a) Underlying causes: structural abnormalities responsible for the weakening of the heart pump.

b) Precipitating causes: specific incidents that, when superimposed on an already weakened heart, will bring on manifestations of heart failure.

The *underlying causes* of congestive heart failure are varied. Heart failure may be due to irreversible damage to the heart muscle from one or more myocardial infarctions (heart attacks). As a result of the damage, the pumping function of the heart becomes impaired, and manifestations of heart failure occur. Heart failure may also be caused by a defective (either "narrowed" or "leaky") heart valve. In such a case, the heart muscle is progressively weakened by the excessive burden imposed by the valvular defect. Finally, heart failure may result from chronic and excessive elevation of the blood pressure, such as in long-standing hypertension.

One or more *precipitating causes* are found in about half of the patients who develop worsening symptoms of congestive heart failure. The most common causes are related to an inappropriate easing of treatment, such as discontinuation of medications, excess of salt intake, or overexertion. This may happen, for example, when a patient with serious underlying heart disease incorrectly assumes that his underlying condition has been "cured," and therefore decides to discontinue or reduce his medications. In some patients, heart failure may be precipitated by the development of other associated conditions (such as cardiac arrhythmias, high blood pressure, anemia, or pregnancy), all of which place an additional burden on the already weakened heart.

The Physiology of Congestive Heart Failure

When an excessive burden upon the heart exists, the body provides some relief in the form of compensatory mechanisms designed to help the ventricles carry on with their pumping function. When the excessive burden is due to an increased pressure load (as with a "narrowed" valve), the result is hypertrophy (thickening) of the ventricular wall, thereby adding to the number of heart muscle units able to contract and strengthening the force of contraction. On the other hand, when the increased burden is caused by excessive volume load (as with a "leaky" valve), the result is dilatation (enlargement) of the ventricle. Through dilatation, the failing ventricle is capable of ejecting an increased amount of blood when it contracts, and is thus able to maintain a normal cardiac performance.

Early in the course of the disease, the compensatory mechanisms are generally adequate to maintain a normal or a near normal cardiac performance. If the excessive burden on the heart persists, however, these mechanisms eventually fail to preserve a satisfactory cardiac function, and manifestations of heart failure may result.

When the weakened left ventricle (main pumping chamber) fails to empty properly, blood returning to it from the lungs backs up and accumulates "upstream," in the left atrium and in the lungs. As a result, the

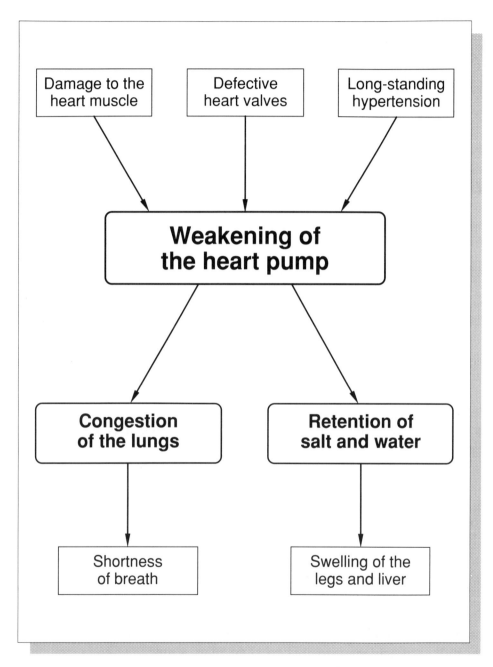

Figure 39. The basic mechanisms of congestive heart failure.

pressure in the left atrium and in the pulmonary (lung) circulation rises. (See figure 39). If the pressure becomes excessive, it will result in leakage of fluid from the tiny capillaries into the lung tissue, a condition termed pulmonary congestion. The presence of fluid in the lung tissue stiffens the lungs and also interferes with the gas exchange, therefore resulting in a sensation of shortness of breath.

When the failing heart is unable to maintain a satisfactory output of blood, the delivery of blood to vital organs, especially the kidneys, is diminished. When the delivery of blood to the kidneys becomes inadequate, this leads to retention of salt and water, through a series of complex mechanisms. This in turn increases the volume of fluids within the body, and ultimately leads to congestion of organs and tissues, especially swelling of the legs and ankles (leg edema), and congestion of the liver.

Symptoms of Heart Failure

Shortness of breath (dyspnea) is the most common symptom of congestive heart failure. The type of dyspnea varies from patient to patient, and depends on the severity of the underlying condition. In patients with mild heart failure, for example, symptoms are usually minimal and occur only during exertion. In patients with moderate or severe heart failure, on the other hand, symptoms are more pronounced and may occur during limited activity or even at rest.

Patients with mild heart failure usually first experience *dyspnea on exertion,* that is, shortness of breath occurring during exercise and physical activity. Patients may report that a specific activity which they were able to carry out without difficulty for many years (such as climbing several flights of stairs) requires them to stop briefly midway because of shortness of breath. As heart failure progresses, the symptoms worsen, and the exercise capacity may decline, over a period of months or weeks.

Another typical symptom of congestive heart failure is *orthopnea,* that is, shortness of breath that develops in the lying position. It is due to the rapid shift of fluids from the lower extremities into the central circulation when the patient lies down. The failing heart is unable to pump the extra volume of blood delivered to it, and the pressure in the pulmonary circulation rises further, leading to increased shortness of breath. The patient with orthopnea often elevates his head on several pillows to prevent difficulty in breathing at night. Sometimes, the patient may be suddenly awakened at night with a feeling of suffocation (paroxysmal nocturnal dyspnea). In advanced cases, symptoms may be so severe that the patient must spend the entire night in the sitting position.

The most dramatic symptom of congestive heart failure is *pulmonary edema,* which results from "flooding" of the alveoli (the tiny air sacs in the lungs) with fluid. In the typical case, the patient suddenly develops severe breathlessness and becomes extremely anxious. He often coughs up a pink, frothy liquid, causing him to feel as if he is literally drowning. The patient is often covered with cold sweat, and his skin is cold and clammy. Pulmonary edema is often a terrifying experience for both patient and bystander. It is a medical emergency, and the patient must be brought to a hospital without delay, for otherwise it may be fatal.

Nonspecific symptoms of heart failure, such as fatigue and weakness, represent poor delivery of blood to the skeletal muscles in patients with poor cardiac function. Some patients with advanced heart failure, especially the elderly, may experience confusion and memory loss, due to poor delivery of blood to the brain. Occasional patients may develop a dry, nonproductive cough, which in this case represents pulmonary congestion.

Guidelines: Recognizing the Symptoms

Notify your physician if you develop any of the following symptoms (especially if you have a history of heart disease):

• You experience increasing breathlessness and fatigue during activities you were able to perform before (such as walking up a flight of stairs, or vacuuming the carpet).

• You begin to gain weight rapidly (more than a pound per day), over a period of several days. Your legs and ankles swell up, and your shoes become tight.

• You require more pillows to sleep at night. You awaken in the middle of the night with a sense of not getting enough air.

Diagnosing Congestive Heart Failure

The diagnosis of congestive heart failure is often suspected in patients with progressive symptoms of shortness of breath and fatigue. The physical examination and diagnostic tests will help confirm the presence of heart failure and assess its severity.

Physical Examination

The general appearance of the patient when seen by the doctor is important. Patients with mild to moderate heart failure, for example, may develop difficulty breathing upon walking a few steps in the doctor's office or while undressing.

During the examination of the lungs, the doctor will auscultate with his stethoscope, listening to the breath sounds during respiration (breathing). In patients with heart failure, the lungs become congested with fluid, and moist crackling sounds (rales) can be heard over the lower portion of the lungs. As heart failure progresses, these rales will become more numerous and will be heard over larger portions of the lungs.

Some patients may develop a collection of fluid between the lungs and the chest wall (pleural effusion). In order to detect this fluid, the doctor will percuss (thump) with his fingers on the patient's back, seeking areas of dullness. The resulting sound is somewhat similar to the sound made by tapping a barrel containing fluid.

The doctor will then listen carefully to the heart sounds. In some patients with a weakened heart, he may hear an abnormal heart sound, called a gallop sound (it resembles a horse's gallop), representing an abnormal function of the heart pump. In others, he may hear a heart murmur, resulting from turbulence in the bloodstream, usually representing a malformed or defective heart valve.

The examination of the lower extremities may reveal leg edema (swelling). Gentle finger pressure at the ankle will often produce a characteristic "pitting" of the fluid-filled soft tissue. The examination of the abdomen may reveal an enlarged liver, due to congestion of the liver tissue. The retention of fluid within the body tissues is usually accompanied by a progressive weight gain, over a period of days or weeks.

Diagnostic Tests

The purpose of diagnostic tests in patients with congestive heart failure is three-fold: confirm the suspected diagnosis; assess the severity of heart failure; and discover the underlying cause of the problem.

The two most useful noninvasive tests in patients with heart failure are the chest x-ray and the echocardiogram. In some patients, additional invasive procedures (such as cardiac catheterization and coronary angiography) will be indicated, in order to obtain more specific and accurate diagnostic information.

The *chest x-ray* is excellent for visualizing the "lung fields," containing the lung tissue and the pulmonary blood vessels. In patients with heart failure, the lungs become congested and fill up with fluid, giving a typical pattern of white patchy areas within the lung fields (pulmonary congestion pattern). In patients with pleural effusion, the chest x-ray can detect the presence of fluid between the lungs and the chest wall. In addition, the chest x-ray can visualize the size and shape of the cardiac silhouette, and is therefore helpful in detecting any abnormal cardiac enlargement, which is often present in patients with long-standing heart disease.

The *echocardiogram* is especially useful in diagnosing the underlying cause of heart failure. It provides detailed information on the function of the heart muscle, the dimensions of the heart chambers, and the condition of the heart valves. The echocardiogram is helpful in differentiating between the various forms of heart disease (such as coronary artery disease, valvular heart disease, congenital heart defects, and heart muscle disease), all of which can lead to manifestations of congestive heart failure.

In selected patients, especially those suspected of having a correctable condition (such as a defective heart valve, a congenital defect, or severely narrowed coronary arteries), additional diagnostic procedures will be indicated. *Cardiac catheterization* allows the measurement of pressures within the heart chambers and pulmonary circulation, and is thus useful in assessing the severity of the heart failure state. Injection of dye into the heart chambers or major blood vessels (angiography) can be performed, in order to assess the function of the ventricles and visualize the heart structures. Finally, *coronary angiography* provides a detailed picture of the coronary arteries, and is thus very useful in showing areas of abnormal narrowing or total blockage in patients with coronary artery disease.

The Management of Congestive Heart Failure

The first step in the management of heart failure is the correction of the precipitating cause. The doctor will try to identify and treat any specific incidents (such as excess of salt intake, cardiac arrhythmias, or elevated blood pressure) that might have brought on the condition. In about half of the cases, however, no precipitating cause will be found.

Another important step is the correction of the underlying cause. The doctor will conduct a thorough examination and will order a series of diagnostic tests, in order to identify and eventually correct the underlying condition. Some patients, in whom the underlying problem is severe hypertension, for example, may benefit from a better control of their condition with antihypertensive drugs. If the problem is correctable only with surgery, however, then an operation may be indicated.

The treatment of the heart failure state is based on the use of three different approaches that complement each other:

a) *Reduction of the heart's workload:* this can be achieved by physical and emotional rest, and weight reduction.

b) *Control of excessive salt and water retention:* this can be accomplished by a low-salt diet, and the use of diuretics.

c) *Improvement of the heart's pumping function:* the medications most often used for this purpose are digitalis drugs and vasodilators.

Physical and Emotional Rest

Restriction of physical activity is important in patients with heart failure. The degree of physical activity allowed can be adjusted to the severity of the patient's symptoms. If, for example, shortness of breath occurs only while the patient is carrying grocery bags or climbing three flights of stairs, he should be advised to make every effort to discontinue those activities. If it is essential for these activities to be continued, they should be carried out more slowly and should be interrupted with rest periods. In obese patients, weight reduction is important, since this will diminish the workload on the heart pump.

Adjustments in lifestyle are often necessary. Strenuous or competitive sports should be discouraged. Golfers, for example, may use a golf cart instead of walking. In patients with more severe symptoms, adjustments in the work schedule are often needed. The working day can be reduced to 5 hours, or the work week reduced to 4 days, with a day of rest during the middle of the week.

In the presence of severe heart failure, hospitalization for several days is often desirable. This facilitates the search for a precipitating cause, and allows adjustment of treatment while the patient is under observation. Hospitalization is also beneficial because it allows a more rigorous control of restricted physical activity, and removes the patient from situations at home and at work that might be emotionally stressful.

Low-salt Diet

In patients with heart failure, considerable improvement in symptoms may result from a simple reduction in salt intake. The normal diet contains about 6 to 10 grams of salt per day. This intake can be cut in half simply by elimination of the salt shaker at the table, and by excluding salt-rich foods such as pretzels, popcorn, salted nuts, potato chips, delicatessen meats, herring, and pickles.

There is usually no need to eliminate the salt in cooking (and make the diet unpalatable), unless fluid retention occurs despite the use of diuretic drugs. The poor taste of a low-salt diet may cause unnecessary hardship to patients and their families and may interfere with adequate nutrition. Only in occasional patients will a strict low-salt diet be necessary.

Drug Therapy

The drugs most commonly used in the treatment of congestive heart failure include the diuretics ("water pills"), the digitalis ("heart pills"), and the vasodilators.

Diuretics. Diuretics are drugs that increase urinary elimination of both salt (sodium chloride) and water. Most diuretics act on the kidneys by blocking the absorption of salt and water by the kidney, thereby increasing urine volume. This results in lessening of fluid retention and edema, and leads to improvement in the symptoms of heart failure. The availability of potent diuretics allows the patient to eat a nutritious and palatable diet, which contains some salt.

The use of diuretics is associated with a number of side effects, some of them potentially serious. All diuretics induce loss ("wasting") of potassium in the urine, thus causing depletion of body potassium. A low potassium level in the blood can in turn result in symptoms of weakness and fatigue, and can sometimes lead to disturbances of the cardiac rhythm. The overuse of diuretics can also result in excessive loss of salt and water, eventually leading to significant weight loss, low blood pressure, and fatigue.

The loss of potassium can be counteracted by eating potassium-rich foods (such as fruits and vegetables), or by taking potassium supplements (liquid or tablets). Some diuretics contain a second drug that prevents loss of potassium; in this case, potassium supplements are usually not necessary (and may be even dangerous), unless prescribed by the doctor.

Digitalis. Digitalis drugs have been used in the treatment of heart failure for over 200 years. They increase the contractility of the heart muscle, and thus improve the performance of the failing heart. The most commonly used digitalis drug is digoxin (Lanoxin®), often referred to as the "heart pill." Digoxin is eliminated from the body very slowly, and is prescribed as a convenient once-a-day dose.

Digitalis drugs are effective, but they must be taken under close medical supervision, since they can result in varied and potentially serious toxic reactions. Excessive amounts of these drugs can accumulate in the body, eventually resulting in digitalis toxicity. The manifestations of digitalis toxicity are varied and nonspecific, and may include nausea and vomiting, drowsiness, and blurred vision. The most dangerous toxic effects, however, are disturbances in the cardiac rhythm, which can be extremely serious. It is important that patients become aware of this potential toxicity and never take more than the amount prescribed.

Vasodilators. These are drugs that relax the peripheral blood vessels, and thus lower the resistance against which the heart must pump. This results in improvement of the cardiac function, reduction of the pressure in the lungs, and relief of the symptoms of heart failure. The vasodilators are potent drugs, but they also have significant side effects, and their use is best reserved for the treatment of severe heart failure, especially when there has been a poor response to optimal doses of diuretics and digitalis.

17 Cardiac Arrhythmias

To carry out its task, the heart depends upon the distribution of tiny electrical impulses that travel from the atria (upper chambers) to the ventricles (pumping chambers). The electrical currents within the heart regulate its rhythm, that is, the coordinated contraction of the atria and ventricles. Disturbances of the heart rhythm, termed cardiac arrhythmias, result from disruption in either the formation or the conduction of these electrical impulses.

The Cardiac Electrical System

The rhythmic contraction of the heart chambers is under the control of the sinus node, a small bundle of highly specialized cells that generate tiny electrical impulses. (See figure 40). The sinus node functions as the "natural pacemaker," setting the pace for the heartbeat. The sinus node is located at the top of the right atrium. From there, the electrical signals spread throughout the atria, causing them to contract and squeeze their blood content into the ventricles.

From the atria, the electrical signals reach the atrioventricular (AV) node, located at the junction of the atria and ventricles. The AV node acts as a relay station and "gateway" to the ventricles. From the AV node, the signals are conducted via the conduction system made of a bundle of specialized muscle fibers (called the bundle of His), which then divides into two branches, called the left and right bundle branches. Each bundle branch divides into a network of smaller fibers which stimulate the ventricles, causing them to contract and pump blood.

Under resting conditions, the heart rate is normally between 60 and 100 beats per minute. The heart rate is mainly dictated by the demands placed upon it. During exercise or excitement, for example, the heart responds to the increased demands by beating faster, thereby pumping more blood. During periods of intense exercise, the heart may speed up to rates of 160 to 200 beats per minute.

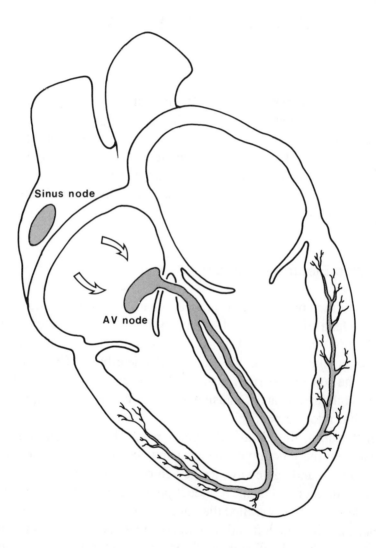

Figure 40. The cardiac electrical system.

Diagnosing Cardiac Arrhythmias

Patients with cardiac arrhythmias may have a variety of symptoms. When the rhythm is irregular, abnormally slow, or abnormally fast, this may cause palpitations — an unpleasant awareness of the beating of the heart. When the heart rate becomes extremely slow or extremely fast, insufficient blood is delivered to the body. This leads to a temporary reduction of blood flow to the brain and may result in symptoms of lightheadedness, dizziness, or syncope (fainting spell).

It should be noted that some patients with significant cardiac arrhythmias may experience no symptoms at all. Vice versa, patients complaining of palpitations, dizziness or fainting spells may have a perfectly regular rhythm. Therefore, diagnostic tests are often necessary to evaluate patients suspected of having cardiac arrhythmias. The most useful tests are the electrocardiogram (ECG) and the ambulatory ECG monitoring (Holter).

The Electrocardiogram (ECG). The ECG is a graphic recording of the electrical activity generated in association with the heartbeat (see also Chapter 9). The ECG tracing is a combination of deflections in sequence representing the electrical events within the heart (figure 41). The P wave is the first small deflection of the ECG, representing the contraction of the atria. The QRS complex, which normally follows the P wave, represents the contraction of the ventricles. By carefully examining the P waves, the QRS complexes, and the sequence of the electrical events on the ECG, the doctor is able to diagnose the vast majority of cardiac arrhythmias.

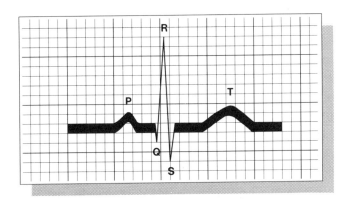

Figure 41. The ECG tracing.

The ECG tracing is useful when an arrhythmia occurs during the period of recording. Quite often, however, the rhythm disturbance is transient (short-lived) and will not occur during the brief period of actual recording (which lasts for less than a minute). Thus, a normal ECG does not exclude the presence of an arrhythmia. If an arrhythmia is suspected, further diagnostic tests may be necessary.

Ambulatory ECG Monitoring (Holter). This is a 24-hour recording of the electrical activity generated by the heart (see also Chapter 9). The patient is instructed to engage in his usual daily activities, and to document in a diary the various activities performed (such as exercise, emotional stress, sexual intercourse) as well as any symptoms (palpitations, dizziness, or faintness) he may experience during the test. The Holter monitoring is extremely useful in detecting intermittent cardiac arrhythmias. It also permits correlation between the time of their occurrence and the patient's recorded activities and symptoms.

General Management of Cardiac Arrhythmias

The primary goal of antiarrhythmic therapy is to restore and maintain a normal rhythm, and prevent the recurrence of arrhythmias. Before initiating therapy, the physician will try and answer several basic questions:

• Is an arrhythmia present? Based on the findings of the ECG and Holter monitoring, the physician is usually able to confirm the presence of an arrhythmia and diagnose its exact nature.

• What is the significance of the arrhythmia? There are multiple causes for rhythm disturbances other than heart disease; these may include drug toxicity, low potassium level, infections, and congestive heart failure. In many of these disorders, treatment of the underlying cause will often eliminate the arrhythmia with no need for any specific antiarrhythmic therapy.

• Does it require treatment? Not every arrhythmia will require treatment! Most antiarrhythmic drugs can cause adverse effects. The decision whether or not to treat is often difficult, and the potential benefit of any treatment must be weighed against its risk.

• What is the most effective and safest treatment? Once the physician has concluded that an arrhythmia should be treated, then the most appropriate means of therapy can be selected.

. . . . . .

Three general modalities are used for the treatment and control of cardiac arrhythmias:

a) Antiarrhythmic drugs, given either intravenously for rapid control of serious arrhythmias, or orally in less urgent situations.

b) Electrical cardioversion (electric shock), used to restore a normal sinus rhythm in the case of certain tachycardias.

c) Artificial pacemaker, used to maintain a satisfactory heart rate during episodes of severe bradycardia or certain types of heart block.

(For further discussion of these treatment modalities, see below)

Common Cardiac Arrhythmias

The normal rhythm is under the control of the sinus node (the "natural pacemaker"), and is therefore termed normal sinus rhythm. During normal sinus rhythm, the heart rate is between 60 to 100 beats per minute, and the rhythm is regular (figure 42).

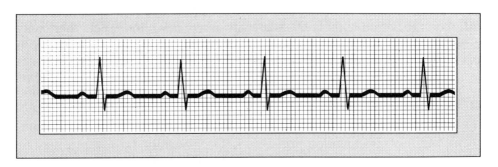

Figure 42. Normal sinus rhythm.

Cardiac arrhythmias result from disturbances in the formation of the electrical impulses within the heart's electrical system. The heart may beat too slowly (under 60 beats per minute), producing bradycardia. Or it may beat too rapidly (over 100 beats per minute), resulting in tachycardia. Other times, the rhythm may become irregular or erratic.

Certain cardiac arrhythmias can occur in the absence of any structural abnormalities of the heart. A number of factors can disturb the heart's normal rhythm, among them cigarette smoking, anxiety, excess caffeine, alcohol, and the use of certain medications. Various cardiac conditions (such as coronary heart disease, valvular disorders, congenital defects) as well as non-cardiac disorders (thyroid disease, lung disease, potassium imbalance) may also result in disturbances of the cardiac rhythm.

Rhythm disturbances can originate anywhere in the cardiac electrical pathway, which extends from the sinus node to the terminal fibers in the ventricles. Depending on the site of origin of the rhythm disturbance (sinus node, atria, or ventricles), the various arrhythmias can be conveniently divided into several subgroups.

Arrhythmias Arising in the Sinus Node

Sinus Bradycardia. The sinus node discharges at a slow rate, less than 60 beats per minute. The rhythm remains regular. In most instances, sinus bradycardia is a benign arrhythmia, which does not necessarily indicate heart disease. In fact, it often occurs in healthy young adults, particularly well-trained athletes. In some cases, however, sinus bradycardia may indicate the presence of a serious underlying problem. It may be seen, for example, in some patients during the early hours after a myocardial infarction (heart attack). If the heart rate slows down too much, there may be excessive reduction of blood flow to the brain, and this may result in symptoms of dizziness or faintness.

Sinus Tachycardia. The sinus node discharges rapidly, at a rate exceeding 100 per minute. The rhythm remains regular. Sinus tachycardia is generally a normal reaction to body "stresses," such as exercise, emotional excitement, and fever (to mention just a few). Occasionally, however, it may be associated with serious underlying conditions, such as heart failure, increased thyroid activity, or anemia. In such cases, treatment must be directed at the underlying condition.

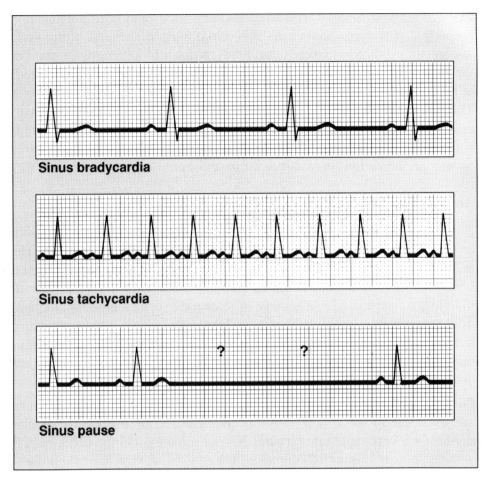

Figure 43. Arrhythmias arising in the sinus node.

Sinus Pause. The sinus node suddenly fails to discharge, resulting in a pause between two successive heart beats. The ECG shows an abnormal pause between two successive P waves. Sinus pause is commonly associated with underlying heart disease, such as coronary heart disease, digitalis toxicity, or the "sick sinus syndrome" (see below). Symptoms of dizziness or fainting will generally occur if the pause lasts for more than 3 to 4 seconds. An artificial pacemaker (see page 207) is usually indicated when symptoms are present.

"Sick Sinus Syndrome." The sinus node is "sick" and does not function properly. The term applies to the coexistence of several sinus node abnormalities, such as marked sinus bradycardia, prolonged sinus pauses, or the alternation of periods of significant slowing of the heartbeat with periods of sudden acceleration (the so-called "bradycardia-tachycardia syndrome"). The sick sinus syndrome is most often seen in patients with coronary heart disease and in the elderly. Patients often complain of symptoms, such as palpitations, dizziness, or fainting spells. The presence of symptoms is usually an indication for an artificial pacemaker.

Arrhythmias Arising in the Atria

Premature Atrial Contractions. There is a premature (early) discharge from an abnormal site in the atrium, occurring before the next expected beat. The ECG tracing shows an early P wave followed by a QRS complex of normal configuration. Premature atrial contractions commonly occur in normal individuals, especially in a variety of situations such as emotional stress, drinking coffee, or smoking cigarettes. They may be associated with almost any kind of heart disease. Premature atrial contractions often cause palpitations, which can be bothersome if frequent. Otherwise, they are usually of little clinical significance, and may not require treatment.

Paroxysmal Atrial Tachycardia ("PAT"). There is rapid discharge from an abnormal site in the atrium. PAT is characterized by a perfectly regular rhythm, at a very rapid rate (around 200 per minute). On the ECG, each P wave is followed by a QRS complex, which is usually of normal configuration. "Paroxysmal" means that the episode ("attack") starts suddenly and then stops suddenly. The episode may last from a few seconds to a few hours. In most patients, the episode is associated with significant palpitations ("racing heart") and anxiety. Occasionally, it may result in dizziness, faintness, or shortness of breath. PAT may be associated with various types of heart disease, but is commonly seen in otherwise healthy individuals. It can be treated and prevented with antiarrhythmic drugs.

Atrial Fibrillation. There is a very rapid and disorganized firing from multiple sites in the atrium. Most stimuli are blocked at the level of the AV node (the "gateway" to the ventricles), but some stimuli are conducted down the conduction pathway and activate the ventricles, thus resulting in an irregular and erratic heartbeat. The ECG tracing shows small irregular waves of the baseline, no P waves, and an erratic ventricular rhythm. Atrial fibrillation is often associated with palpitations, and occasionally may cause dizziness or shortness of breath. It is generally seen in association with various types of heart disease, but may also occur in persons with a normal heart. Atrial fibrillation can be "paroxysmal" (recurrent) or "chronic" (persistent). The paroxysmal type can be prevented with antiarrhythmic drugs. In patients with the chronic type, the heart rate can be slowed down with certain drugs (such as digitalis).

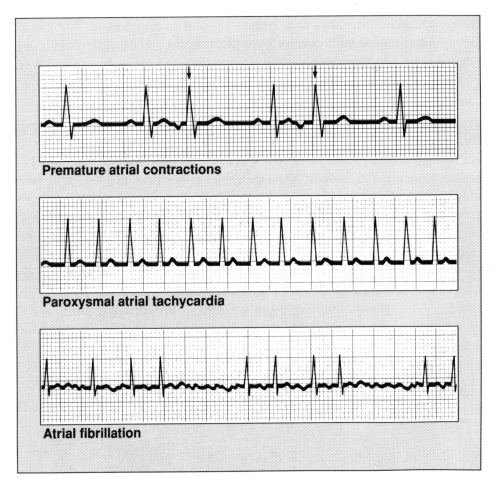

Premature atrial contractions

Paroxysmal atrial tachycardia

Atrial fibrillation

Figure 44. Arrhythmias arising in the atria.

Arrhythmias Arising in the Ventricles

Premature Ventricular Contractions (PVCs). They result from an irritable site in the ventricles. When the irritable site discharges, the result is a beat that occurs prematurely (early), before the next expected beat. The ECG shows a wide QRS complex of bizarre configuration, occurring early, before the next expected QRS complex. The PVC is usually followed by a brief pause, often described by the patient as a "skipped beat" sensation. The beat that follows the PVC is usually more forceful than a regular beat, therefore often causing a "flip-flop" sensation in the chest. PVCs commonly occur in individuals with no heart disease, especially in association with emotional stress, smoking cigarettes, or drinking coffee. They also occur in association with various types of heart disease, especially coronary heart disease. In the absence of underlying heart disease, the presence of PVCs is usually of no major concern.

Ventricular Tachycardia. It results when an irritable site in the ventricles discharges repetitively at a fast rate. The ECG shows a rapid succession of PVCs, giving the appearance of a series of wide undulations (wavy lines). An episode usually lasts for a few seconds, but occasionally may last for several minutes. When brief, the arrhythmia may cause no symptoms, or it may be associated with palpitations, often described as a "fluttering" sensation in the chest. When sustained, especially if the rate is rapid, ventricular tachycardia can cause symptoms of dizziness and syncope (fainting spell). Ventricular tachycardia is a serious arrhythmia, and is almost always indicative of significant underlying heart disease. It is frequently seen in the early hours following a myocardial infarction (heart attack). Ventricular tachycardia can be treated with drugs given into the vein, or with emergency electrical cardioversion. It can be prevented with antiarrhythmic drugs taken orally.

Ventricular Fibrillation. This is a chaotic rhythm that results when multiple irritable sites in the ventricles start firing at an extremely rapid rate. The ventricles are unable to respond completely and effectively to each stimulation, and as a result there is a very rapid, irregular, uncoordinated "twitching" of the ventricles. The ECG shows a rapid and totally irregular rhythm, with bizarre patterns of varying size and configuration. Ventricular fibrillation is the most serious arrhythmia that exists, and it is equivalent to cardiac arrest. There is no pulse and no breathing, and the patient loses consciousness within a few seconds. If the normal rhythm is not restored promptly with resuscitation and electric shock (defibrillation), death follows within a few minutes. Ventricular fibrillation is most commonly seen in patients with severe coronary heart disease, especially during the first few hours after an acute myocardial infarction (heart attack). It is the most frequent underlying rhythm leading to sudden cardiac death.

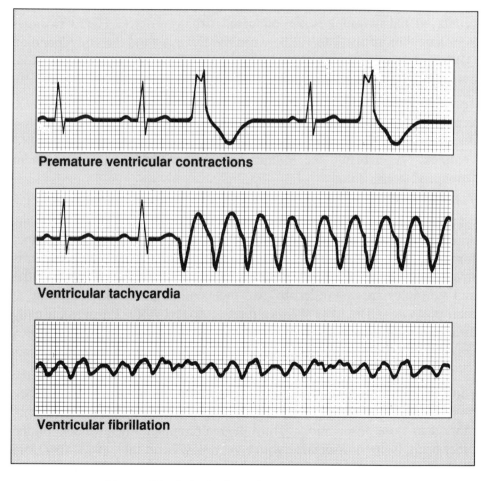

Figure 45. Arrhythmias arising in the ventricles.

Heart Block

Heart block (or AV block) is caused by disruption of the electrical conduction pathway somewhere between the atria and the ventricles, usually at the level of the AV node. As a result of the block, there is a temporary delay or a total interruption of the impulse conduction between the atrial impulse and the eventual ventricular response.

The various types of heart block can be classified into three categories, in order of increasing severity:

First-degree heart block. The conduction between the atria and ventricles is delayed, but all impulses are conducted to the ventricles. The ECG shows a prolongation of the interval between the P waves and the corresponding QRS complexes. The rhythm remains regular, however, and there is no evidence of "dropped" beats.

Second-degree heart block. Most of the atrial impulses are conducted to the ventricles but some are not. Periodically, the atrial impulse fails to stimulate the ventricles. On the ECG, some P waves are not followed by a QRS complex. As a result, the rhythm becomes irregular, with intermittent "dropped" beats.

Third-degree (complete) heart block. There is complete interruption of the conduction pathway, and all atrial impulses are blocked. The ventricles are stimulated by a secondary "safety pacemaker," located within the conduction pathway below the block site. The rate of the secondary pacemaker is much slower than the primary pacemaker (sinus node). As a result, the atria and ventricles are controlled by two independent pacemakers, beating at their own rates. The ECG shows a regular atrial rhythm (P waves), usually at a rate above 60 per minute, and a regular ventricular rhythm (QRS complexes) at a much slower rate, usually under 40 per minute.

The severity of the heart block is highly variable and depends on the clinical circumstances. Most cases of first and second-degree heart block do not cause any symptoms and usually do not require any special treatment other than close observation. Third-degree (complete) heart block, on the other hand, is often associated with a very slow heart rate, and is therefore likely to cause significant symptoms, such as fatigue, lightheadedness, and recurrence of fainting spells. Patients with complete heart block and a slow heart rate are usually candidates for an artificial pacemaker.

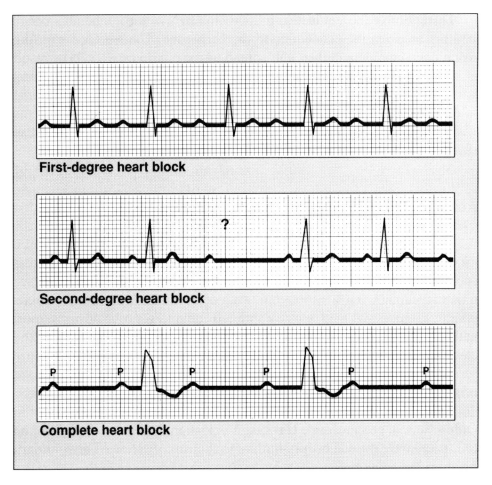

First-degree heart block

Second-degree heart block

Complete heart block

Figure 46. Types of heart block.

Heart block can be "chronic" (long-lasting) or "transient" (temporary). Chronic heart block is commonly seen in patients with coronary heart disease, in whom the conduction system has been damaged by a previous myocardial infarction. It is also frequently seen in the elderly, the result of a degenerative process involving the conduction system. Transient heart block is most often associated with a fresh myocardial infarction. Other times, it may result from excessive dosage or toxicity of certain antiarrhythmic drugs, such as digitalis.

Disruption of the conduction in *either* the right *or* the left bundle branch will not interrupt the conduction to the ventricles. The stimulus will first reach one ventricle and then will spread to the other ventricle. The result is a *bundle branch block*. Bundle branch block is usually seen in patients with various types of heart disease (especially coronary heart disease) and in the elderly. Occasionally, a bundle branch block can be seen in patients with a normal heart. Since it does not cause any disturbance in the cardiac rhythm, bundle branch block does not cause any symptoms.

Antiarrhythmic Drugs

Numerous agents are available for the treatment of cardiac arrhythmias. (See also Chapter 22). There is generally more than one way to treat a specific arrhythmia, but there is usually one drug that is the most effective one for that particular situation ("the drug of choice"). Most drugs are quite effective, but they may also cause side effects. In excessive dosages, most antiarrhythmic drugs will cause some degree of toxicity, especially on the cardiovascular system. Some antiarrhythmic drugs, for example, can cause serious cardiac arrhythmias, which may be even more dangerous than the original arrhythmias for which the drug was initially prescribed!

Three antiarrhythmic agents, quinidine (brand names: Quinidex®, Quinaglute®), procainamide (Pronestyl®, Procan SR®), and disopyramide (Norpace®) have a somewhat similar mechanism of action. Their primary action is the suppression of the irritable discharging sites in the ventricles or atria. These drugs are used primarily in the treatment and prevention of premature ventricular contractions and ventricular tachycardia. They are also effective in the control of certain atrial arrhythmias.

Digitalis drugs, such as digoxin (Lanoxin®), in addition to their use in the treatment of congestive heart failure, are quite effective in the management of certain cardiac arrhythmias. As antiarrhythmic agents, their main action is to slow down the transmission of atrial impulses through the AV node (the "gateway to the ventricles"), thus slowing down the rate at which the ventricles beat. In patients with chronic atrial fibrillation, for example, a daily dose of digitalis is useful in slowing down and controlling the heartbeat. Taken on a daily basis, they are also effective in preventing the recurrence of several other atrial arrhythmias.

The beta blockers, such as propranolol (Inderal®), are used in the treatment of several arrhythmias (they are also effective agents for treating angina and hypertension). The beta blockers act by blocking the action of adrenaline on the beta receptors in the heart. The result is a slowing of the heart rate, as well as a reduction in the force of cardiac contraction. Their main use as antiarrhythmic agents is in slowing the ventricular rate in certain atrial arrhythmias. They are not as effective as digitalis for this purpose, and are often used as a drug of second choice, either alone, or in combination with digitalis. The beta blockers are sometimes useful in preventing the recurrence of ventricular arrhythmias, especially those associated with emotional stress and exercise.

During certain emergency conditions (such as following a fresh myocardial infarction), arrhythmias may be dangerous, and even life-threatening, if not treated promptly. In such circumstances, drugs need to be given intravenously (into the vein), so they can start acting immediately. Lidocaine, for example, when given intravenously, is very effective in suppressing ventricular arrhythmias, such as frequent premature ventricular contractions and ventricular tachycardia.

In the setting of a fresh myocardial infarction, marked sinus bradycardia may cause significant slowing of the heartbeat, and may lead to deterioration of the patient's condition. Atropine, given intravenously, is usually effective in increasing the rate of the sinus node, thus improving the cardiac performance. When sinus bradycardia is excessive, however, or when it is caused by a complete heart block, atropine may not be effective, and the insertion of a temporary pacemaker may be necessary.

Electrical Cardioversion

Electrical cardioversion is an electric shock delivered through the chest wall, used in the treatment of certain rapid tachycardias. The shock causes electrical discharge of the entire heart simultaneously, temporarily "wiping out" all electrical activity. This allows the sinus node to resume its normal function as the dominant pacemaker.

During the procedure, two round paddles are positioned over the patient's chest. To prevent the skin from being burned, the paddles are coated generously with a special electrode paste. The patient is given a brief general anesthesia, with an anesthetic agent injected into the vein. Once the patient is asleep, the physician checks the position of the paddles, and then delivers an electric shock through the chest wall. The patient's response usually consists of a single twitch of the chest muscles, or a slight jerk of the arms. The procedure is not painful, and most patients do not have any memory of the event. If the initial low-energy shocks do not cause electrical discharge of the heart, successive shocks can be delivered without delay at increasing energy levels until cardioversion is achieved.

Emergency cardioversion is performed in certain urgent situations, when there is a need for prompt treatment of serious or life-threatening arrhythmias. Generally, most ventricular and atrial tachycardias can be controlled with antiarrhythmic drugs (given intravenously or orally). When associated with a very rapid heart rate, however, these tachycardias can severely compromise cardiac performance, and may lead to a significant drop of blood pressure and loss of consciousness. A typical example is the cardioversion of ventricular tachycardia during the early stages of fresh myocardial infarction. If not treated promptly, this serious arrhythmia may cause rapid deterioration in the patient's condition, and may lead to ventricular fibrillation and death.

As we have seen, ventricular fibrillation is the most dangerous arrhythmia that exists, and it is equivalent to cardiac arrest. If a normal rhythm is not restored immediately, death follows within a few minutes. An emergency electric shock (called defibrillation) is the only effective treatment for ventricular fibrillation, and it must be done promptly, otherwise the chances for survival are dismal.

Elective cardioversion ("elective" meaning non-urgent) is used in the treatment of certain chronic cardiac arrhythmias, when there is no need to terminate the arrhythmia right away. A typical example is the elective cardioversion of chronic atrial fibrillation. Cardioversion is quite an effective technique, and it will restore a normal sinus rhythm in the majority of the patients treated. The result, however, is often not sustained for long periods. In fact, fewer than half of the patients with chronic atrial fibrillation will remain in sinus rhythm one year following cardioversion. Thus, it is the maintenance in a normal sinus rhythm which is the difficult problem, and not the immediate termination of the arrhythmia.

Artificial Pacemakers

When the sinus node (the "natural pacemaker") does not function properly, or when the conduction pathway is disrupted, the heart may beat too slowly (bradycardia). An excessively slow heartbeat can cause a temporary decrease of blood flow to the brain, and may result in symptoms of lightheadedness, dizziness, or fainting spells. In many cases, this may be remedied by the implantation of an artificial pacemaker, which takes over for the sinus node (the "natural pacemaker") during periods of excessive slowing of the heartbeat. Pacemakers were first successfully implanted during the 1960s, and since then, hundreds of thousands of pacemakers have been implanted worldwide.

The pacemaker is an electronic device that delivers electrical stimuli to the heart. It consists of two basic parts: a pulse generator and a pacing wire (see figure 47). The pulse generator is composed of a battery which supplies energy for the stimuli, and an electronic circuit that regulates the electrical impulses that are sent to the heart. The pacing wire is an insulated, flexible wire that conducts the electrical stimuli to the heart muscle. The wire has two functions: it carries impulses from the pulse generator and relays them to the heart ("pacing" function); it also senses signals from the heart and relays them to the pulse generator ("sensing" function).

Two general types of pacemakers are available. The simpler type, the "fixed-rate" pacemaker, puts out electrical impulses continuously at one preset rate (usually 70 per minute), whether or not the heart is beating on its own. The more sophisticated "demand" pacemaker senses the heart's natural rhythm and emits impulses to stimulate the heart only when the natural heart rate falls below the pulse-generator's set rate (usually 60 or 70 per minute). In other words, this type of pacemaker works only when it is needed, when the natural rhythm is too slow. The demand type pacemaker is the one most commonly used at the present time.

A temporary pacemaker is used in the management of transient (short-lived) bradycardias, such as those seen in the setting of a fresh myocardial infarction, or in association with drug toxicity. It is utilized in a hospital setting (usually in the coronary care unit), for a period of several days, until the arrhythmia has subsided. A permanent pacemaker, on the other hand, is indicated when the bradycardia is likely to be chronic or recurrent. It is implanted permanently in the patient's body.

Indications For a Pacemaker

Artificial pacemakers are used in the treatment of marked bradycardias, when the excessive slowing compromises the pumping function of the heart, or when the slowing results in significant symptoms.

The most common indication for a pacemaker is a complete heart block. There is a disruption of the conduction pathway somewhere between the atria and the ventricles, and as a result, the ventricles beat at a very slow rate (often under 40 beats per minute). Patients often experience symptoms of fatigue, dizziness and fainting spells. The treatment of complete heart block with drugs is usually ineffective and unreliable. The use of a pacemaker is often the only way to keep the heart rate at a satisfactory level.

Another frequent indication for a pacemaker is the presence of the "sick sinus syndrome." As we have seen, the term applies to the existence of several sinus node abnormalities, including marked sinus bradycardia, prolonged sinus pauses, and the alternation of periods of very slow and very fast heartbeat (the so-called "bradycardia-tachycardia syndrome"). Patients may complain of recurrent symptoms, such as palpitations, dizziness, or fainting spells. Most patients with the sick sinus syndrome, especially those having symptoms, will require insertion of a pacemaker.

Temporary Pacemakers

Temporary pacing is indicated in cases of severe bradycardia, when it is felt that the arrhythmia is transient (short-lived). In fresh myocardial infarction, for example, the slowing of the heart is often transient, and improves within a few hours or days. In such circumstances, the insertion of a temporary pacemaker can prevent the occurrence of marked slowing of the heartbeat during the critical period. The pacing wire will be then removed once the condition has improved.

The insertion of a temporary pacemaker is usually performed in the emergency room or in the coronary care unit (CCU). The procedure is done at the patient's bedside, using local anesthesia. The pacing wire is inserted through a vein in the upper chest or through a vein in the arm. The wire is then directed into the right ventricle, following the path of blood returning to the heart. A portable x-ray machine is helpful in guiding the pacing wire and positioning it in the heart.

After the pacing wire has been positioned properly, its connector end is attached to the pulse generator, which is about the size of a small transistor radio. The pulse generator is left outside the patient, and in this way the physician can easily regulate the heart rate when it becomes necessary. Once the arrhythmia has improved, and the danger of marked slowing of the heart beat is over, the pacing wire is removed by the physician. If the arrhythmia persists for several days with no improvement, however, then a permanent pacemaker may be indicated. The insertion of a temporary pacemaker is relatively simple, takes about an hour or two, and usually causes minimal pain or discomfort.

Permanent Pacemakers

Permanent pacing of the heart is indicated in patients who have a marked bradycardia associated with symptoms, when the bradycardia is likely to be permanent or recurrent. The permanent pacemaker is actually implanted inside the patient's body, to stay there permanently.

Today's pacemakers are highly sophisticated electronic devices. Advances in technology have enabled pacemakers to become considerably reduced in size. A modern permanent pacemaker is small, thin, and lightweight, about the size of a pocket watch. This makes the pacemaker more convenient for the physician to "implant," and more cosmetically attractive to the patient. Along with reduction in size, the longevity of pacemakers has been dramatically increased. The pacemaker's power source is a long-life battery that is hermetically sealed, along with the circuitry, inside the pulse generator. The estimated life of a modern pacemaker is about eight to ten years.

Most modern permanent pacemakers are "programmable," that is, one or more of their parameters (such as rate) can be adjusted from the outside, without surgery. The physician, through the use of an electronic device placed outside the patient's body, can send electronic signals to the pacemaker. Thus, it is possible to alter the pulse generator's operation to fit changes in the patient's needs. Reprogramming is a simple procedure that can be done within minutes at the doctor's office or clinic.

Some cardiac conditions respond best when the electrical impulses are transmitted to both the atria and ventricles, in sequence. The sophisticated "AV sequential" pacemaker is especially designed for such conditions. This

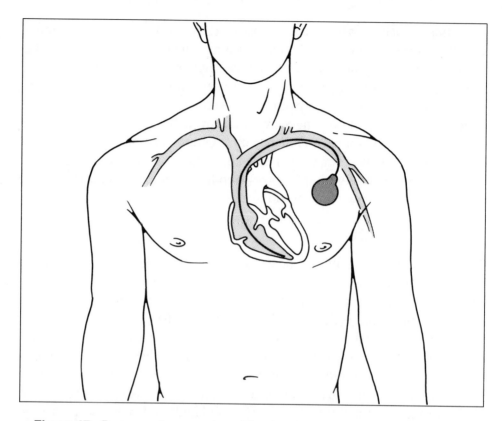

Figure 47. Permanent pacemaker. The tip of the pacing wire is inside the heart. The pulse generator is placed outside the chest, under the skin.

technique uses two pacing wires, one positioned in the atrium and the other one in the ventricle, and both are connected to the pulse generator. The advantage of AV sequential pacing is a better coordination between the contraction of the atria and ventricles, and therefore a somewhat better cardiac performance. The AV sequential pacemaker is more difficult to install and is more expensive compared to the standard demand pacemaker. Therefore, it is best reserved for selected patients who will benefit from its special features.

The implantation of a permanent pacemaker is generally performed in the operating room, under local anesthesia. The physician (cardiologist or chest surgeon) prepares the implantation site by cleansing and anesthetizing the upper chest area below the collarbone. An incision is made to expose a vein. The pacing wire is then introduced into the vein, and directed toward the heart, while the physician watches its progress on a television screen. Next, a small "pocket" is created in the area of the incision. The connector end of the wire is plugged into the pulse generator, which is then inserted into the pocket. The incision is sutured closed and bandaged, and the patient returns to his room. The procedure takes about two hours, and is associated with only minimal pain or discomfort.

Following the implantation of the pacemaker, patients are usually kept in the hospital for a few days. Even though the pulse generator may feel a little uncomfortable at first, most patients eventually become accustomed to it, and are able to go back to work, travel, bathe, exercise, and in general, live normal and active lives. Contrary to what some patients may think, however, a pacemaker will not cure the underlying heart condition and will not make the heart stronger!

Pacemaker Follow-up

Despite the reliability of modern pacemakers, they are subject to potential malfunctions. Causes for pacemaker malfunction may include displacement of the pacing wire, fracture of the pacing wire, and failure of the pulse generator. These problems may result in failure of the pacing function, sensing function, or both.

It is therefore very important that the pacemaker performance be checked on a regular basis. The doctor may do this in person, or he may refer the patient to a pacemaker clinic. Generally, the pacemaker should be checked at intervals of 3 to 6 months. In some patients, telephone monitoring of the pacemaker function can be performed; using a special transmitter, the patient can transmit an ECG tracing directly to the doctor's office or to the pacemaker clinic. Checking the pacemaker this way is convenient, but is not a substitute for regular medical checkups.

Most modern pacemakers are equipped with special circuitry that is resistant to electrical interference. Therefore, it is unlikely that anything in the usual home environment will interfere with the pacemaker's function. Generally, modern microwave ovens should not damage the pacemaker or interfere with its function. However, certain industrial areas or certain devices may be a potential source of strong electrical interference. These may include electrical power plants, an industrial environment with electric arc welders, radio or television transmitters, and certain medical diagnostic or therapeutic devices. For this reason, patients should be aware of any environments or devices that could affect their pacemaker's function.

Following discharge from the hospital, the patient receives a pacemaker I.D. card, which supplies basic information about the pacemaker, and provides the name of the physician. The I.D. card can be a lifesaver in case of serious illness, accident, or pacemaker malfunction. The card should be carried by the patient at all times.

18 Sudden Cardiac Death

Sudden death can be defined as an unexpected death, from natural causes (therefore excluding homicide, accidents, poisoning, and suicide), occurring within minutes of the onset of the terminal event. Sudden death may result from a wide variety of causes (respiratory, neurological, or metabolic), but in the vast majority of cases it is due to a sudden collapse of the cardiovascular system.

In the industrialized nations, sudden cardiac death constitutes about 20 percent of all natural fatalities. In the United States, for example, as many as 450,000 persons succumb to this condition each year (nearly one death every minute!). Sudden cardiac death is 3 to 4 times more common in men than in women.

The Mechanisms of Sudden Cardiac Death

In the majority of patients who die suddenly, the underlying mechanism is a primary electrical failure of the heart. The cause of death is most often ventricular fibrillation, a chaotic rhythm that results when multiple irritable sites in the ventricles start firing at a rapid rate. The ventricles are unable to respond effectively to each stimulus, and the result is a very rapid, irregular, uncoordinated "twitching" of the ventricles. In a small number of patients, electrical failure is due to asystole, that is, a complete absence of contractions of the ventricles.

Both ventricular fibrillation and asystole are equivalent to cardiac arrest: there is no pulse and no breathing, and the patient loses consciousness within a few seconds. If the cardiac rhythm is not restored promptly with resuscitation measures, death follows within a few minutes.

The overwhelming majority of sudden deaths are related to impaired delivery of blood to the heart muscle in patients with extensive coronary artery disease. Among these patients, about 20 percent of sudden death cases appear to be related to an acute myocardial infarction (heart attack). In most other cases, sudden death is associated with a temporary impairment of blood flow to the heart muscle (ischemia). The temporary ischemia results in "starving" of the heart muscle for oxygen, increased irritability of the ventricles, and increased vulnerability to electrical failure.

When sudden cardiac death develops as a consequence of an acute myocardial infarction, the event is often preceded by symptoms, such as chest pain, profuse sweating, nausea, shortness of breath, or weakness. Death most commonly occurs within the first two hours after the onset of symptoms, often before the patient is able to reach the hospital. In these patients, the mechanism for sudden death is either an electrical failure (ventricular fibrillation or asystole) or a mechanical failure (massive infarction or rupture of the heart).

When ventricular fibrillation occurs in the setting of an acute myocardial infarction and the patient is successfully resuscitated, the recurrence of such an event is rare and the prognosis is generally good. In fact, the life expectancy in these patients is essentially the same as in patients with comparable infarctions who had not experienced ventricular fibrillation.

Although coronary heart disease accounts for the great majority of sudden cardiac deaths, a wide variety of other cardiac conditions have been implicated, including congenital defects, valvular disease, and heart muscle disease. Rare cases of sudden death have also been reported in people with normal hearts, presumably as a result of primary electrical failure.

Approaches to the Problem of Sudden Cardiac Death

Because most victims of sudden death die outside a hospital, doctors have tended to consider it as a complex problem over which they had no control. However, with the advent of coronary care units (CCUs), the extensive use of ECG monitoring, and the widespread popularization of cardiopulmonary resuscitation (CPR) techniques, it has become increasingly clear that many cases of sudden cardiac death were reversible, if treated in time. This realization has led to renewed efforts to identify those individuals who may be at risk of sudden death, and to take appropriate preventive actions.

There are essentially two approaches for containing the problem of sudden cardiac death. The first approach is a community-wide educational program of CPR. The major limitations of this approach relate to the fact that the victim is often reached only after the event, and even a trivial delay or minor errors in technique can spell failure. In addition, even the most successful outcome provides no assurance against recurrence.

The second approach is the identification of patients who are most susceptible to ventricular fibrillation, and initiation of preventive anti-arrhythmic therapy before the event. Studies have shown, for example, that the presence of frequent or complex premature ventricular contractions (so-called "malignant" PVCs) in patients with severe coronary artery disease is associated with an increased risk of ventricular fibrillation and sudden cardiac death. The mere presence of PVCs (even if frequent) in patients with a normal heart, however, does not appear to increase the incidence of sudden cardiac death.

Patients who were resuscitated from an episode of sudden cardiac death have a high risk of a repeat episode (except when the episode has occurred in the setting of an acute myocardial infarction). In such patients, specialized invasive techniques (such as electrophysiological studies) are often indicated, in order to assess the nature of the underlying cardiac arrhythmia and find an appropriate preventive therapy.

Electrophysiological studies are sophisticated and complex invasive techniques, performed in selected patients suspected of having potentially life-threatening arrhythmias. During the test (which is performed in the "cath lab") special catheter-electrodes are introduced through the veins and directed toward the heart under x-ray control. These electrodes are then used to stimulate different portions of the heart muscle, in order to detect increased irritability and predisposition to arrhythmias. Several antiarrhythmic drugs are then tested. Drugs that can end these artificially induced arrhythmias are likely to prevent the recurrence of future attacks of ventricular fibrillation and sudden cardiac death.

Cardiopulmonary Resuscitation (CPR)

Cardiac arrest (from either ventricular fibrillation or asystole) is followed within a few seconds by respiratory arrest and loss of consciousness. The clinical state of unconsciousness associated with lack of ventilation or circulation is referred to as cardiopulmonary arrest.

The victim in cardiopulmonary arrest is in imminent danger of permanent, irreversible damage to the brain, from lack of oxygen (hypoxia). If hypoxia is relieved within 3 to 5 minutes, recovery is generally complete. However, hypoxia exceeding 4 to 6 minutes usually causes severe and permanent injury to the brain.

The aim of cardiopulmonary resuscitation (CPR) is to establish ventilation and circulation that will provide adequate oxygen delivery to vital organs, particularly the brain. It requires learning the skills of artificial respiration ("mouth-to-mouth" breathing) and closed chest compressions ("cardiac massage"), as well as the proper timing and specific sequence in which to use these steps.

The CPR sequence begins when one comes across an apparently unconscious victim. The "rescuer" must first determine whether the victim is indeed unconscious or merely sleeping. He must then be sure that the airway (the passage between the mouth and the lungs) is not blocked by the tongue, which would prevent the victim from breathing. Then he must determine if the victim is breathing, and if there is a pulse (indicating circulation). If the unconscious victim is found not breathing and without pulse, the rescuer should then start mouth-to-mouth breathing and chest compressions.

Remember!

Written material alone does not constitute a CPR course! It is necessary to practice on manikins (dummies), under the guidance of certified instructors, to gain the skills of CPR. It is strongly recommended that those who wish to learn CPR take a formal course (offered by the American Heart Association or the American Red Cross), which will allow adequate time to practice under close supervision.

Basic Guidelines for CPR

1) Establish Unresponsiveness and Call for Help

When you come across a seemingly unconscious victim, you must first establish unresponsiveness. Tap the person on the chest and shout: "Are you OK?." If you get no response, shake the person gently by the shoulders and shout again. At the same time, call out for help and summon bystanders. For CPR to be effective, the victim must be flat on his back on a firm surface. If you find the victim lying face down, you will have to turn him over. Support his neck and head with one of your hands as you turn him.

2) Open the Airway

Once the person is on his back and you are sure he is unconscious, you must open the airway to be sure that he can breathe. In an unconscious person, the tongue relaxes and falls against the back of the throat, preventing air from getting from the mouth and nose to the lungs. When the neck is extended, the tongue pulls away from the back of the throat, opening the airway. In order to extend the neck, place one hand over the victim's forehead, and put your other hand under his neck to support it. Then push down and back on his forehead with one hand, while gently lifting up his neck with the other hand. This "head-tilt maneuver" will open the airway in most victims. This technique should not be used in persons with suspected neck injury.

3) Check for Breathing

With your hands still in place, check for breathing. Looking toward the victim's chest, bend over so that your cheek is almost touching his nose and mouth. *Look* to see if his chest is rising and falling, *listen* for sounds of breathing, and *feel* expired air on your cheek. Look, listen, and feel for several seconds.

Continued

4) Give 4 Quick Breaths

If there is no evidence of breathing, the victim is not getting any oxygen, and you want to get as much oxygen into him as possible. Keep your hands in place on his forehead and neck to keep the airway open. Then, using the hand on his forehead, pinch his nostrils together tightly with your thumb and forefinger to keep air from escaping through his nose. Take a deep breath, open your mouth wide, and place it completely over the victim's mouth to make a tight seal with your lips. Exhale into the victim's mouth 4 times, in rapid succession. Take your mouth away to inhale between breaths, but do it quickly so that the victim's lungs don't completely empty between the breaths. Although you will feel some resistance from the victim's lungs, you should be able to feel air going in as you blow and to see the chest rise and fall.

5) Check for Pulse

Once you have given 4 quick breaths, check to see if the victim has a pulse. The easiest pulse to check is located on either of the carotid arteries, which run down both sides of the neck. Keeping your other hand on the forehead, take your hand from under the victim's neck and place 2 fingers on his Adam's Apple. Then slide them over into the groove between the Adam's Apple and the neck muscle on the side closer to you. The carotid pulse should be felt in the space between these structures. If you don't find the pulse immediately, move your fingers around slightly. Allow adequate time (5 to 10 seconds); the pulse may be slow, or very weak and rapid.

6) Get Help

If a second person is present, now is the time to have him or her call for help. Send someone to call 911 or your local emergency number. This will activate the Emergency Medical Services (EMS) system. If you are still alone, perform CPR for at least 1 minute before stopping to call EMS yourself.

Continued

The EMS system includes an efficient communication alert system, well trained rescue personnel who can respond rapidly, ambulances that are properly equipped, and emergency facilities that are open 24 hours a day to provide advanced life support.

7) Rescue Breathing

If the victim is not breathing, you must start artificial ventilation ("mouth-to-mouth"). Just as you did before, keep your hands in position on the neck and forehead, pinch the nostrils closed, inhale and make a seal with your mouth, and exhale air into the victims lungs. Between breaths, turn your head to the side and look, listen, and feel for the victim's breathing. Do it once every 5 seconds, taking your mouth away between breaths. If there is no pulse, you must provide artificial circulation (provided by external chest compression) in addition to rescue breathing.

8) Chest Compression

If there is no pulse, you will have to create artificial circulation of the blood by compressing and releasing the chest. By pushing down on the chest, you are squeezing the heart between the breastbone (sternum) and the back bone (spine), thus forcing blood out through the aorta and toward the brain and other vital organs. The heart valves prevent the blood from flowing in the "wrong" direction. Upon release, the pressure in the heart chambers falls, and the heart fills up with blood.

To perform chest compression ("cardiac massage") properly, kneel next to the victim's chest. Locate the notch at the lowest portion of the breastbone and place two fingers on the notch. Place the heel of the other hand next to the fingers, then place your other hand on top of the first. To avoid any injury to the ribs, only the heel of your hand should touch the chest. Shift your weight forward until your shoulders are directly over your hands, and your elbows are straight. Now, bear down and come up, keeping your elbows locked.

Continued

In order to squeeze the heart and circulate the blood, you must depress the chest about 1.5 to 2 inches (for the average adult). The rate of compression should be 80 per minute. To get the proper speed and rhythm, count out loud as you do the compressions: "one-and-two-and-three-and-four-and-five-and...". The compression phase should be equal to the relaxation phase between compressions (approximately half a second each).

Single-rescuer CPR. If you are the only rescuer, you must provide both rescue breathing and chest compression. After each 15 compressions, take your hands off the chest, place them on the neck and forehead as before, pinch the nostrils, seal the mouth, and give 2 strong breaths. Then go back to the chest, find the correct hand position, and do 15 more compressions, followed by 2 breaths. Repeat this cycle of 15 and 2 for a total of 4 times, which will be about 1 minute. Then check again for pulse and breathing. If there is no pulse, resume CPR. If there is a pulse but no breathing, apply rescue breathing only. You must continue chest compressions and rescue breathing until the patient revives, qualified help comes, or you are too exhausted to continue.

Two-rescuer CPR. If there is another rescuer to help you, position yourselves on opposite sides of the victim. One rescuer is responsible for compressing the chest, at a rate of 60 compressions per minute. To get the proper speed and rhythm, count out loud as you do the compressions: "one-thousand-two-thousand-three-thousand-four-thousand-five-thousand...". The other rescuer is responsible for interposing a breath during the relaxation of each fifth compression, giving a compression/breath ratio of 5 to 1. Once every few minutes, the rescuers may switch roles. The switch must be performed quickly and smoothly to maintain effective CPR.

CPR on Children and Infants

The steps of CPR and the sequence in which they are performed remain the same as in adults. Modifications have been made, however, to compensate for the smaller body size.

Continued

CPR on children (1 year to 8 years): For chest compressions, use only one hand. Depress the chest 1 to 1.5 inches with each compression. To get the proper speed and rhythm, count out loud as you would for an adult: "one-and-two-and-three-and-four-and-five-and...". Give 1 breath for every 5 compressions.

CPR on infants (up to 1 year): For rescue breathing, cover and seal both the infant's nose and mouth with your mouth. Give gentle "puffs" of breath. Since the carotid pulse is difficult to locate on infants, use the brachial pulse on the inside of the arm, midway between the elbow and the shoulder. If there is no pulse, begin chest compressions by placing your index finger and middle finger on the middle of the breastbone and depressing no more than 1/2 to 1 inch. Compression rate should be 100 per minute. Count out loud as you do the compressions: "one-two-three-four-five....". Give one gentle breath every 5 compressions.

It should be emphasized, once again, that written material alone does not constitute a CPR course! It is necessary to practice on manikins, with certified instructors, to gain the skills of CPR.

19 Valvular Heart Disease

The heart valves are flexible structures that regulate the flow of blood within the heart. A diseased or defective valve interferes with the normal one-way flow of blood as it is pumped through the heart. As a result, the heart must pump harder in order to compensate for the poorly functioning valve. Eventually, the overworked heart becomes unable to sustain the burden, and symptoms develop.

Understanding Valvular Disease

Heart valves function like one-way doors, allowing the blood to circulate in only one direction, and preventing it from backing up (figure 48). The valves possess either two or three leaflets (or cusps). They open and close depending upon the force of blood within the heart chambers. (For more information on how the heart works, see Chapter 6).

A normal heart valve is flexible enough to open and permit blood to flow through it, yet strong enough to hold back the flow when closed. A defective valve is one that fails to either open or close fully. *Stenosis* of a valve is its inability to open fully ("narrowed" valve), thus delaying forward blood flow. The result is backup of blood and increased pressure in the heart chamber located upstream to the narrowed valve. *Regurgitation* (or *insufficiency*) of a valve is its inability to completely close ("leaky" valve), thus permitting leakage of blood in the "wrong" direction. With the next heartbeat, the regurgitated blood must again flow through the valve, together with the normally flowing blood. As a result, the heart chamber involved must pump harder to handle a larger volume of blood.

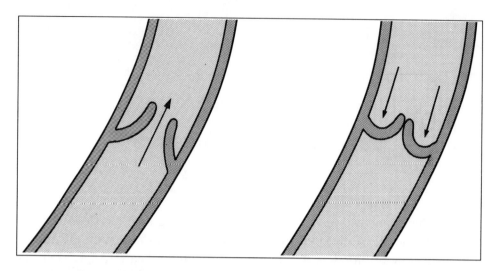

Figure 48. The valves allow the blood to circulate in only one direction, and prevent it from backing up.

When the pumping function of the heart becomes impaired as a result of a defective heart valve, the body itself provides some relief in the form of *compensatory mechanisms,* which are designed to help the ventricles carry on their function.

When the aortic valve becomes narrowed, for example, this results in an increased pressure load on the left ventricle. Compensation is obtained from hypertrophy (thickening) of the ventricular muscle, thereby adding to the number of heart muscle units able to contract, and strengthening the force of contraction. (See figure 49).

When the aortic valve is "leaky," on the other hand, the result is an excessive volume load on the ventricle. The body response is generally a dilatation (enlargement) of the ventricular chamber. Through dilatation, the ventricle is capable of ejecting an increased amount of blood when it contracts, and is thus able to maintain a satisfactory cardiac function.

Early in the course of valvular disease, the compensatory mechanisms are capable of maintaining a normal or near normal cardiac performance. With time, however, valvular defects gradually tend to get worse. Eventually, the compensatory mechanisms fail, and symptoms develop.

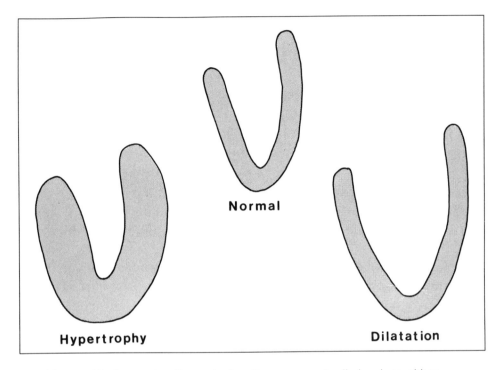

Figure 49. Long-standing valvular disease eventually leads to either hypertrophy or dilatation of the heart chambers.

Causes of Valvular Disease

The most common type of valvular disease is *rheumatic heart disease,* which results from rheumatic fever (see below). It is characterized by a progressive scarring and deformity of the heart valves, leading to variable degrees of valvular stenosis (narrowing) and regurgitation (leakage). Although greatly diminished since the advent of antibiotics, rheumatic heart disease still affects nearly two million Americans living today.

Valvular disease can also be caused by *congenital valvular defects,* that is, valvular defects present at birth (see Chapter 20). These defects result from aberrant development of the valvular structures in the fetal heart. The cause for the malformation is only rarely identified. In fact, the cause of the congenital defect remains unknown in over 90 percent of cases.

Another common cause for valvular dysfunction is *degenerative valvular disease,* which is most frequently seen in the elderly. The valvular defect is caused by the aging process and by the wear and tear of the valvular structures. Over the years, the soft and pliable valvular tissue becomes more rigid. In some patients, the valvular tissue may also become calcified, that is, hardened by deposits of calcium. The degenerative process may interfere with the normal function of the valve, and may lead to narrowing or leakage of the valve. Degenerative valvular defects most commonly involve the aortic and mitral valves, probably because of the higher pressure and increased wear and tear in the left side of the heart.

Sometimes valvular damage can be caused by *infective endocarditis,* that is, infection of the heart valves (see Chapter 21). Infective endocarditis most commonly occurs in patients who already have pre-existing valvular defects. The condition is caused by bacteria that have entered the bloodstream and settled on the heart valves. If the circumstances are favorable for infection, the bacteria grow and multiply and eventually form cauliflower-like growths, called vegetations. These bacterial growths, which vary in size, interfere with the valvular function, and may sometimes destroy part of the valvular tissue. The result is an improper closure of the valve, and therefore leakage of the valve.

Rheumatic Fever

Rheumatic fever is an inflammatory disease that affects the connective tissue in various parts of the body, especially in the joints and the heart. The primary victims of rheumatic fever are children between the ages of five and fifteen. Once a widespread, crippling, and even life-threatening disease, rheumatic fever is now relatively rare. This is due mostly to a more effective diagnosis and early antibiotic treatment of the initial infection.

An attack of rheumatic fever can usually be traced to an upper respiratory infection ("strep throat") that had occurred and cleared up two or three weeks earlier. Typical manifestations of "strep throat" include a sudden onset of symptoms, a sore throat, swollen glands in the neck, and high fever. When a child develops these symptoms, a throat culture is generally taken. If the culture shows the presence of streptococcus (a type of bacteria), treatment with antibiotics is begun and continued for about ten days. If treatment is not given, rheumatic fever may follow.

In some children, the antibodies (produced by the immune system to combat the streptococcus bacteria) may erroneously attack the connective tissue of the joints and the heart, eventually causing rheumatic fever. The child with rheumatic fever generally develops symptoms of fever, fatigue, and poor appetite. Several joints may become tender and swollen. If the heart is involved, the child may develop a heart murmur, an enlarged heart, or manifestations of heart failure. Frequently, however, children who have involvement of the heart do not have any symptoms referable to the heart, and the condition may not be diagnosed at that time.

Although rheumatic fever generally strikes children, the manifestations of rheumatic heart disease do not become apparent until years later. The initial damage to the valve is the result of inflammation during the episode of rheumatic fever. During the healing process, which takes months and often years, scar tissue may cause portions of the affected leaflets to partially fuse together, thus resulting in deformity of the valve. The leaflets tend to fuse along the natural lines of their closure (commissures). (See figure 50). The gradual scarring of the valves eventually leads to variable degrees of valvular narrowing (stenosis) or leakage (regurgitation).

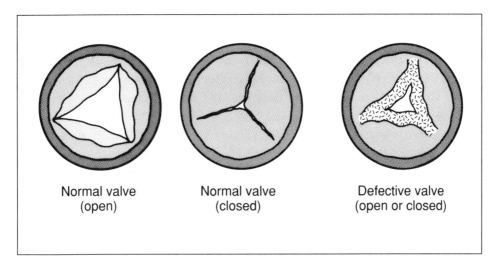

| Normal valve (open) | Normal valve (closed) | Defective valve (open or closed) |

Figure 50. In rheumatic valve disease, scar tissue causes portions of the leaflets to fuse together, leading to deformity of the valve.

Common Types of Valvular Disease

Diseases of the heart valves are classified according to the specific valve involved and the type of valve defect. The most common valvular abnormalities are: mitral stenosis, mitral regurgitation, aortic stenosis, and aortic regurgitation. Valvular diseases involving the tricuspid and pulmonic valves are rather uncommon, and will not be discussed in this chapter.

Not infrequently, there may be involvement of two valves (usually the mitral and aortic valves) in the same patient. Other times, there may be a combination of both stenosis and regurgitation of the same valve. The clinical diagnosis of such complex valvular abnormalities is often difficult, and generally requires the skills of a well-trained cardiologist.

Mitral valve prolapse is a common condition which results from a defect of the mitral valve. Because of its peculiarities and characteristic clinical manifestations, it will be discussed separately (see page 239).

Mitral Stenosis

In the majority of cases, mitral stenosis is caused by rheumatic heart disease. During the healing process following rheumatic fever, scar tissue causes portions of the mitral valve leaflets to partially fuse together, generally along their natural lines of closure (commissures). The scarring process leads to the gradual narrowing of the valve. The narrowed mitral valve is typically funnel-shaped, and the opening (orifice) is frequently shaped like a "fish mouth" or buttonhole. Over the years, there is thickening of the valve leaflets as well as deposits of calcium, causing the valve to become thickened and rigid.

The narrowing of the mitral valve slows down the free flow of blood from the left atrium to the left ventricle. Blood returning from the lungs backs up in the left atrium and in the lungs. As a consequence, there is a gradual increase of the pressures in the left atrium and in the pulmonary (lung) circulation. The constant elevation of pressure in the left atrium leads to the gradual dilatation of that chamber. When the pressure in the lungs becomes excessive, it may result in leakage of fluid from the tiny capillaries into the lung tissue (pulmonary congestion). The presence of fluid in the lung tissue stiffens the lungs and interferes with the gas exchange, often resulting in a sensation of shortness of breath.

The initial bouts of shortness of breath in patients with mitral stenosis are usually precipitated by exercise, emotional stress, or infection (all of which increase the flow of blood and result in further elevation of the pressure in the lungs). As the condition progresses, the symptoms worsen, and the exercise capacity gradually declines.

In patients with advanced mitral stenosis, the left atrium gradually enlarges. As the atrial walls continue to stretch, the weakened atrium may be unable to contract normally, and atrial fibrillation may develop (see page 198). In atrial fibrillation, there is erratic "quivering" of the atrial walls, and the contraction of the atrium is ineffective. The onset of atrial fibrillation often causes further deterioration of the patient's condition, since the already weakened atrium is now unable to propel blood efficiently.

Mitral Regurgitation

In about half of the cases, mitral regurgitation is caused by rheumatic heart disease. Following an episode of rheumatic fever, there is progressive scarring of the mitral valve, with rigidity, deformity, and retraction of the mitral leaflets. As a result, the mitral valve does not close tightly, and some of the blood flows backward into the left atrium during the contraction of the left ventricle. In patients with rheumatic heart disease, the scarring and deformity of the mitral leaflets often cause both narrowing and leakage, and thus often result in combined mitral stenosis and regurgitation.

Mitral regurgitation can also be caused by a defect of the mitral valve apparatus present at birth (congenital). Other times, it may follow disruption of the mitral valve structures later in life, either from a degenerative process in elderly persons, or following a myocardial infarction (heart attack). Occasionally, the disruption of the mitral valve is caused by an infection of the valve (infective endocarditis). Another important cause of mitral regurgitation is mitral valve prolapse, a condition characterized by an abnormal stretching and elongation of one or both mitral leaflets, resulting in an oversized or "floppy" valve (see page 239).

Normally, during ventricular contraction (systole), the aortic valve opens and blood is forced under pressure into the aorta. At the same time, the mitral valve snaps shut, thus preventing blood from flowing back into the left atrium. In mitral regurgitation, as a result of the valvular defect, the mitral valve leaflets do not close tightly (a "leaky" valve), and some of the blood flows backward into the left atrium. With the next heartbeat, the regurgitated blood must again flow through the mitral valve, together with the normally flowing blood. As a result, both the left ventricle and left atrium must pump harder in order to handle the large volume of blood.

During the early stages of mitral regurgitation, compensatory mechanisms are put into action. There is a progressive enlargement of the left atrium. At the same time, there is a gradual dilatation of the left ventricle. Through dilatation, the ventricle is able to eject an increased amount of blood when it contracts, and is thus able to maintain a normal or near normal cardiac function.

Over the years, there is a gradual weakening of the overworked left ventricle. In advanced cases of mitral regurgitation, the left ventricle is unable to handle the large volume of blood. As a result, there is backup of blood in the left atrium and in the lungs, and therefore a progressive elevation of the pressure in the lungs. When the pressure in the pulmonary circulation becomes excessive, pulmonary congestion ensues, and symptoms of heart failure develop. The initial symptoms are usually mild and occur only during exertion or stress. As with mitral stenosis, the symptoms gradually worsen and occur with less and less activity.

Aortic Stenosis

In children and young adults, aortic stenosis is usually the result of a congenital defect. In many of these patients, the aortic valve has only two cusps (so-called "bicuspid" aortic valve) instead of the normal three. Even though the narrowing may be minimal at birth, over the years the valve tends to become rigid and calcified (with deposits of calcium), and this leads to progressive narrowing of the valve orifice.

In adults, aortic stenosis is most frequently associated with rheumatic heart disease. The healing process following rheumatic fever leads to scarring and fusion of the valvular cusps, and progressive narrowing of the aortic valve orifice. Over the years, there is additional thickening of the cusps as well as deposits of calcium, thus causing the valve to become thickened and rigid. Rheumatic aortic stenosis is generally associated with rheumatic involvement of the mitral valve.

In the elderly, aortic stenosis usually results from a degenerative involvement of the valve. This is due to the aging process and the wear and tear of the valvular structures. Over the years, the cusps become more rigid and deposits of calcium may form on the valvular tissue. The deposits of calcium interfere with the normal function of the cusps, and may lead to the narrowing of the valvular orifice.

The primary abnormality in aortic stenosis is the narrowing of the aortic valve orifice, which leads to slowing of blood flow across the valve during the period of ventricular contraction. In order to eject sufficient blood across the narrowed valve, the left ventricle must develop higher pressures, thus creating a "pressure gradient" (difference of pressure) between the left ventricle and the aorta. The compensatory mechanism for a chronically elevated pressure load is ventricular hypertrophy (thickening), thereby adding to the number of heart muscle units able to contract.

Aortic stenosis may exist for years without producing any symptoms, because the thickened ventricle is usually able to generate enough pressure to maintain a normal or near normal cardiac function. Over the years, however, the narrowing becomes tighter, and the left ventricle may not be able to handle the higher and higher pressure load. As a result, there is backing up of blood in the left atrium and in the lungs, and this eventually leads to pulmonary congestion and symptoms of heart failure.

About half of the patients with severe aortic stenosis will develop recurrent chest pain or discomfort (angina). In these patients, angina results from the inadequate oxygen supply to the markedly thickened and over-worked heart muscle. In some patients with aortic stenosis, angina may also result from coexisting coronary artery disease.

Some patients with severe aortic stenosis will experience symptoms of syncope (fainting spells). Such episodes typically occur during exertion or when the patient stands suddenly. During exertion, for example, there is a sudden increase in the body's demand for blood and oxygen. Because of the severe narrowing of the aortic valve, the heart is temporarily unable to pump sufficient blood to vital organs. This results in a sudden reduction of oxygen supply to the brain, and temporary loss of consciousness.

Aortic Regurgitation

Aortic regurgitation is most commonly caused by rheumatic heart disease. The initial inflammation associated with rheumatic fever leads to progressive deformation and retraction of the aortic cusps. The deformation prevents correct apposition of the cusps and may result in improper closure of the valve. Occasionally, aortic regurgitation occurs in patients with a congenital defect of the valve, such as a bicuspid valve; the defective valve is subject to constant wear and tear, and eventually becomes leaky.

A variety of conditions can produce aortic regurgitation by causing a marked dilatation of the "aortic root" (the portion of the aorta near the heart), without involving the valve directly. As a result of the dilatation of the aortic root, the valvular ring (which supports the cusps) also dilates, the aortic cusps separate, and regurgitation may result. Another cause of aortic regurgitation is infective endocarditis, a bacterial infection that disrupts a portion of the valve tissue.

Normally, the aortic valve opens during the contraction phase of the ventricle (systole), when blood is ejected under pressure into the aorta. During the relaxation phase (diastole), the aortic valve closes, thus preventing blood from flowing back into the ventricle. In aortic regurgitation, the defective valve does not close properly, and some of the blood in the aorta leaks back into the left ventricle. With the next heartbeat, the regurgitated blood must again flow through the valve, together with the normally flowing blood. Even though the amount of blood ejected into the aorta with each heartbeat is larger than normal, a significant portion of it will flow back into the ventricle.

As a result of the leakage, the left ventricle must pump harder in order to handle the large volume of blood. The compensatory mechanism for this excessive volume load is dilatation of the ventricle. Through dilatation, the left ventricle is capable of ejecting a larger volume of blood when it contracts, and thus is able to maintain a satisfactory cardiac function. In chronic aortic regurgitation, there is a slow and progressive deterioration of the function of the left ventricle, over a period of years. When the ventricle finally "fails," blood backs up in the left atrium and in the lungs, eventually leading to pulmonary congestion and symptoms of heart failure.

In patients with chronic aortic regurgitation, there is a long period (often more than 20 years) during which the left ventricle gradually enlarges, while the patient remains symptom-free or nearly so. Patients with severe aortic regurgitation often complain of an uncomfortable awareness of the heartbeat, due to the pounding of the dilated heart against the chest wall. These symptoms may persist for many years before the development of more significant symptoms, such as progressive shortness of breath.

Diagnosing Valvular Disease

Patients with valvular disease can develop a variety of symptoms, such as progressive shortness of breath, palpitations, chest pain, or fainting spells. The physical examination often provides important clues regarding the nature of the defect, and the presence (or absence) of associated congestive heart failure. Diagnostic tests are used to confirm the suspected diagnosis, and to assess the severity of the condition.

Symptoms

Early in the course of valvular disease, the compensatory mechanisms are adequate to maintain a normal or near normal cardiac function. In fact, most patients do not experience any symptoms for a period of years. Eventually, however, the valvular damage gets worse, and the burden on the heart increases. The compensatory mechanisms fail to maintain a satisfactory cardiac performance, and symptoms start to appear.

Patients with significant valvular disease often develop progressive symptoms of shortness of breath (dyspnea) as a result of pulmonary congestion. Initially, symptoms are mild and occur only during physical activity (dyspnea on exertion). As the disease progresses, symptoms become more severe and occur at lower levels of activity, or when lying down at night (orthopnea).

Patients with valvular disease may also experience a variety of other symptoms, such as palpitations, chest pain, or fainting spells (syncope). Palpitations are usually caused by cardiac arrhythmias (disturbances of the cardiac rhythm), which can be seen with almost any type of valvular disease. Patients with aortic regurgitation often complain of an uncomfortable awareness of the heartbeat, usually due to the excessive pounding of the overworked heart.

Chest pain (angina) occurs occasionally, especially in patients with severe aortic stenosis, and is due to insufficient blood supply to the markedly thickened heart muscle. As in patients with coronary heart disease, the pain typically occurs during physical activity or emotional stress and is relieved at rest. Episodes of syncope ("fainting spells") occasionally occur in patients with severe aortic stenosis, especially during exercise or upon sudden standing.

Physical Examination

The most informative step is the examination of the heart. Using his stethoscope, the doctor will auscultate (listen) over several areas of the chest. The normal heart sounds ("lub, dub... lub, dub...") result from the sudden closure of the heart valves during the various phases of the cardiac cycle. Abnormal heart sounds (such as "gallop", "click", and "snap") may represent either a defective valve or weakness of the heart pump.

Heart murmurs result from turbulence in the bloodstream, and usually (but not always) represent a defective valve. Normally, the blood flows silently as long as the flow is smooth. If it has to pass through a narrow orifice at high speed, the flow becomes turbulent, producing a whooshing sound (murmur) that can be heard with a stethoscope. Heart murmurs can occur with either a narrowed valve or a leaky valve. The characteristics of the murmur (such as its timing during the cardiac cycle, its location on the chest wall, or its pitch quality) provide the physician with information regarding the particular valve involved and the type of defect.

As part of a general physical examination, the doctor will also search for signs of congestive heart failure. For example, he will auscultate the lungs with his stethoscope, listening to the breath sounds. In patients with heart failure, the lungs become congested, and crackling sounds (rales) can be heard over the lower portion of the lungs during breathing. He will then examine the abdomen, especially the liver, which may become congested and enlarged in case of significant heart failure. Finally, he will inspect the lower extremities for the presence of leg swelling (edema), which is often (but not always) a manifestation of heart failure.

Diagnostic Tests

Following the medical history and physical examination, if valvular heart disease is suspected, the physician may order a series of diagnostic tests. Most patients will require at least two basic tests: an electrocardiogram (ECG) and a chest x-ray. If further information is needed, the physician may order an echocardiogram, a noninvasive test that can provide accurate information about the heart structures. Finally, in patients with significant valvular disease and progressive symptoms, a cardiac catheterization procedure may be recommended.

The *electrocardiogram (ECG)* is useful in assessing the presence of chamber dilatation (enlargement), which is often found in patients with long-standing valvular disease. Enlargement of the left atrium, for example, often results in typical widening of the P wave. Hypertrophy or dilatation of the left ventricle, on the other hand, results in increased size of the QRS complex. Although useful in detecting enlargement or hypertrophy of specific cardiac chambers, the ECG is not very helpful in assessing the severity of the problem.

The *chest x-ray* is a useful test for the assessment of chamber dimensions in patients with valvular disease. The four chambers of the heart always occupy the same relative position within the "cardiac silhouette." Enlargement of a particular chamber will affect the contour of the cardiac silhouette in a characteristic way, thus helping the physician to identify the chamber involved. The chest x-ray is also useful in assessing the presence of heart failure; when the lungs fill up with fluid and become congested, they may show a typical pattern of white patches within the lung fields (pulmonary congestion pattern).

The *echocardiogram* is extremely valuable in the diagnosis of valvular disease. This sophisticated technique can actually visualize the shape and motion of the heart valves, and detect the presence of valvular defects, such as thickening, calcification, stenosis, and regurgitation. In addition, it can provide detailed information about the dimensions of the heart chambers and the thickness of the ventricular walls. In patients with mitral stenosis, the echocardiogram may even estimate the actual size of the valvular orifice with reasonable accuracy.

Employing these noninvasive tests, the diagnosis of valvular disease will be confirmed in most patients. In some cases, however, invasive procedures will be indicated in order to obtain additional information.

Cardiac catheterization is an invasive technique that provides additional information in patients with significant valvular disease. During the procedure, a thin and flexible plastic tube (catheter) is inserted into a peripheral blood vessel and then directed, under x-ray guidance, toward the heart. (See Chapter 10). Using this technique, the physician can measure the actual pressures within the heart chambers, and the "pressure gradient" across the heart valves (the difference of pressure on both sides of a valve). By injecting dye into the heart chambers (angiogram), the physician can visualize the structures within the heart, including the heart valves. In patients with a leaky valve, for example, the injection of dye within the heart will show a regurgitant flow in the "wrong" direction.

(In most adult patients, a coronary angiogram will be performed in combination with the cardiac catheterization, in order to rule out the presence of significant coronary artery disease).

The decision to perform a cardiac catheterization must be based upon a careful balance between the risks from the procedure and the potential value of the information obtained. Cardiac catheterization is generally recommended when there is a need to confirm the presence of a suspected valvular disease and to define its severity. This need most commonly arises when it is felt that the patient may benefit from cardiac surgery. In general, cardiac catheterization is carried out in all patients for whom a cardiac operation is considered.

Management of Valvular Heart Disease

Patients with no symptoms or minimal symptoms often remain stable for years. In these patients, medical treatment can reduce the symptoms and slow down the progression of the disease. Once symptoms become more severe, however, deterioration may progress rapidly, eventually leading to irreversible damage to the heart muscle and other vital organs.

Medical Treatment

Patients known to have valvular disease may be prescribed preventive antibiotics (prophylaxis) prior to and following certain dental and surgical procedures. This is done in order to prevent the occurrence of infective endocarditis, a condition resulting from bacterial infection of the heart valves (see Chapter 21). This type of infection is more likely to occur following certain dental and surgical procedures during which there is a release of bacteria into the bloodstream. Bacteria have a tendency to lodge on the defective valve and cause endocarditis. Procedures that may require preventive antibiotic treatment include routine dental work, dental and oral surgery, and a variety of procedures involving the respiratory, gastrointestinal, urinary, and genital tracts.

Patients with known valvular disease should be advised to report the development of any new symptoms to their doctor. Generally, they should be cautioned to avoid vigorous physical or athletic activities. In some patients, the condition can worsen progressively without causing new symptoms. Therefore, patients suspected of having a significant valvular defect but no symptoms should be followed carefully by their physician, at regular intervals. They may also need periodic diagnostic tests in order to detect any deterioration of the condition.

Once clinical manifestations of congestive heart failure develop, treatment is initiated (see Chapter 16). Although the treatment may vary depending on the type of valvular disease and its severity, the general principles are the same. In order to reduce the heart's workload, patients are advised to get adequate physical and emotional rest, and to adjust the degree of their physical activity to the severity of their symptoms. Excessive salt and water retention can be controlled with a low-salt diet, and with the use of diuretic drugs. In some patients, the cardiac performance can be improved by the use of digitalis drugs. Although most symptomatic patients will improve with medical treatment, those with progressive symptoms of heart failure despite treatment should be considered for surgery.

Surgical Treatment

The most critical decision in the management of patients with valvular disease concerns the timing of surgery. Patients with valvular disease who have no symptoms or only minimal symptoms are usually not considered for surgery, since they may live for years with little change in their condition. Patients with valvular disease and significant symptoms, on the other hand, may develop irreversible damage of the heart muscle.

The critical time for valve surgery is when the disease has progressed to the point that it may soon result in irreversible damage to the pumping ability of the heart. If surgery is performed before the heart muscle is irreparably damaged, then the outlook is generally good.

A routine cardiac catheterization (with or without a coronary angiogram) is performed in all adult patients who are potential candidates for surgery. This is done in order to confirm the presence of valvular disease, to assess the severity of the condition, and to detect any other unsuspected abnormalities. If both the clinical evaluation and the results of cardiac catheterization suggest that valve surgery could significantly improve the patient's condition, then the decision to operate is made.

The purpose of valve surgery is to replace or repair heart valves that do not function properly. The most commonly used type of surgery is valve replacement, during which the natural but defective valve is replaced with an artificial (prosthetic) valve. The most commonly used valves are the mechanical valves (such as the caged-ball valve and the disc valve), and the tissue valves. (See figure 51).

The caged-ball valve, whose function is somewhat similar to that of a ball valve on a snorkel tube, permits blood to flow freely when the ball is raised and prevents the backward flow when it is dropped. The tilting-disc valve is made of metal and cloth. The disc permits free flow of blood when open and prevents leakage when it flips shut. The mechanical valves have an excellent record of durability, up to 15 or even 20 years. The problem, however, is that blood clots tend to build up on the valve apparatus. For this reason, patients with mechanical valves are routinely prescribed long-term anticoagulant medications (blood thinners).

The tissue (porcine) valve is taken from the heart of a pig and is then chemically treated for use in humans. This type of valve has a low incidence of blood clot formation, since there are no exposed metal parts. Therefore, their use usually does not require blood thinners. Their durability, however, is not as good as the mechanical valves. Tissue valves usually begin to deteriorate after a period of 8 to 12 years, eventually making a second operation necessary.

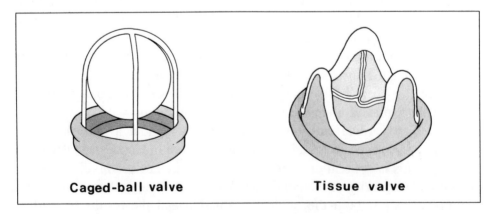

Caged-ball valve   **Tissue valve**

Figure 51. Types of artificial (prosthetic) valves.

Choosing between a mechanical valve and a tissue valve in a particular patient is sometimes difficult. In general terms, a mechanical valve is the more desirable one in relatively young patients who have no contraindications for the use of blood thinners. On the other hand, a tissue valve is often recommended in patients in whom long-term anticoagulant treatment may be hazardous: patients who are prone to bleeding, women who may become pregnant, the elderly, or any patients who appear unreliable or unwilling to take blood thinners on a regular basis.

In selected cases of mitral or aortic stenosis, when the valve is not severely deformed, the surgeon may perform a valve repair. In one type of procedure, termed commissurotomy, the surgeon attempts to free the tight leaflets by separating them at their lines of closure (commissures). This is done by simply spreading (or splitting) the leaflets with the finger, or by cutting the leaflets apart with a surgical knife. Commissurotomy gives the best results in children and young adults, in whom the valve leaflets are still pliable and flexible.

In many respects (other than the actual excision and replacement of the valve), valvular surgery is essentially similar to coronary bypass surgery. Therefore, to learn more about cardiac surgery (such as the preparation for surgery, the operating room, the postoperative period, etc.), the reader is referred to the discussion on coronary bypass surgery, Chapter 24.

Mitral Valve Prolapse

Mitral valve prolapse is the most common abnormality of the heart valves, affecting as many as 5% of adults. This is a variable condition that has attracted considerable attention because of its interesting and peculiar clinical manifestations. It has also generated a lot of controversy as to its clinical significance. In fact, some authorities have speculated that, in the majority of cases, mitral valve prolapse may be simply a normal variant of valve structure rather than "heart disease."

The basic defect in mitral valve prolapse is a structural abnormality of the mitral valve, which leads to an abnormal stretching and elongation of one or both mitral leaflets. Normally, during ventricular contraction (systole), both leaflets snap shut, and their free edges close tightly together, preventing blood from flowing back into the left atrium. In patients with mitral prolapse, the oversized and "floppy" leaflet does not close properly, and prolapses (slips back) toward the atrium (figure 52).

When the mitral leaflet prolapses, it often generates a loud snapping sound (like the sound of a large sail suddenly tensing in the wind), termed a "click." Because of the incomplete closure of the valve there is often, in addition, some leakage of blood toward the left atrium, resulting in turbulence and a heart murmur.

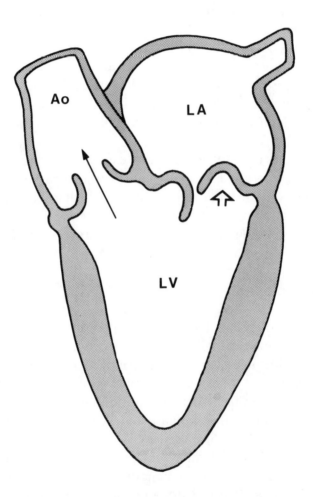

Figure 52. Mitral valve prolapse. During systole, the floppy mitral leaflet does not close properly, and prolapses toward the left atrium.

Clinical Manifestations

Mitral valve prolapse has been observed in patients of all ages and in both sexes. It is most frequently diagnosed, however, in young women. The overwhelming majority of patients do not experience any significant symptoms, and the prolapse is usually discovered during a routine physical examination. It is important to emphasize that mitral valve prolapse is generally a benign condition, and most patients will remain free of symptoms for their entire lives.

The most common symptoms is chest pain, believed to be secondary to the tensing of certain valvular structures during the prolapse. Although quite variable, the pain is typically prolonged, recurrent, not related to activity, and often associated with brief attacks of sharp stabbing pains. Other common symptoms include palpitations and dizziness. The palpitations, often described as "skipped beats" or "racing heart," may be caused by cardiac arrhythmias (disturbances of the heart rhythm). Frequently, however, no arrhythmias are found.

Patients with mitral valve prolapse often suffer undue anxiety and apprehension, perhaps worsened after being informed by the doctor of the presence of "heart disease." Some patients describe "attacks" of multiple symptoms occurring simultaneously, such as chest pain, palpitations, dizziness, fatigue, and anxiety. Reassurance by the doctor that these episodes do not signal imminent cardiac catastrophe is often sufficient to alleviate most of the symptoms.

There is an increased incidence of cardiac arrhythmias in patients with mitral valve prolapse, probably because of the increased irritability of the heart muscle. The most frequently observed arrhythmias are premature ventricular contractions (PVCs), and paroxysmal atrial tachycardia. Even though these arrhythmias often cause troublesome symptoms (palpitations and dizziness), they are usually of a benign nature.

In rare instances, patients with mitral valve prolapse may develop more significant problems. Some patients, for example, may develop a gradual worsening of the valvular leakage, leading to progressive mitral regurgitation. Others may develop infective endocarditis, that is, a bacterial infection of the defective valve. Infective endocarditis can generally be prevented by the use of preventive antibiotics (prophylaxis) prior to certain dental and surgical procedures (see page 275).

Diagnosing Mitral Valve Prolapse

Auscultation (listening) with a stethoscope is extremely useful in the diagnosis of mitral valve prolapse. The abnormal motion of the prolapsing mitral leaflet during systole often results in a loud sound, termed systolic click, generated by the sudden tensing of the mitral valve structures during systole. The click is often followed by a late-systolic murmur, which represents the leakage of blood through the incompletely closed mitral valve. The presence of either a systolic click or a late-systolic murmur is suggestive of the diagnosis. The combination of these two findings in a particular patient is practically diagnostic of the condition.

The *echocardiogram* plays a key role in the diagnosis of mitral valve prolapse. The common finding on the M-mode echocardiogram is the sudden prolapse (displacement) of the mitral valve during systole. In some patients, it gives a typical configuration, termed "hammocking," because of its resemblance to a hammock. The two-dimensional technique is useful in visualizing the displacement of the mitral leaflet(s) toward the left atrium. The degree of prolapse is variable, and there is no clear-cut transition between "normal" and "diagnostic" findings. When the findings are not definite, the echocardiographic interpretation may state: "questionable," "borderline," "mild," or "suggestive of" mitral valve prolapse.

To complicate matters, some patients with typical findings on cardiac auscultation may have a normal echocardiogram and, vice versa, some patients with a normal auscultation may have suggestive findings on the echocardiogram. The acceptance of only the echocardiographic criteria or only the auscultation criteria may result in an over-diagnosis of the condition. In fact, it is not uncommon for patients to be told by one physician that they do have mitral valve prolapse, then to be told by another physician that they do not have it! Such confusion can induce considerable anxiety and may even undermine the confidence the perplexed patient has in any of the involved physicians.

The other noninvasive tests are not useful in the diagnosis of mitral valve prolapse per se, but are often used to diagnose associated conditions. The ECG, for example, is useful in diagnosing associated cardiac arrhythmias. In patients with recurrent palpitations or dizziness, an ambulatory ECG recording (Holter monitor) is useful in the detection of intermittent arrhythmias. In patients with symptoms of chest pain, an exercise stress test (treadmill) is occasionally helpful in excluding the presence of angina and coronary artery disease. It should be mentioned, however, that patients with mitral valve prolapse occasionally have a "false positive" stress test, that is, an abnormal test in the absence of underlying coronary artery disease.

Management of Mitral Valve Prolapse

As we have seen, the diagnosis of mitral valve prolapse is "borderline" in many cases. It is therefore important for the physician not to make a firm and definite diagnosis of this condition, when the findings are equivocal. It is often tempting to use the diagnosis of mitral valve prolapse as an explanation for a wide variety of nonspecific and vague cardiac symptoms (such as chest pains, palpitations, dizziness and fatigue). However, informing the patient that he has "heart disease" may lead to undue anxiety and worsening of the symptoms. The most important aspect of therapy in mitral valve prolapse is reassurance. The physician must explain to the patient the generally benign nature of the condition, and the excellent outlook in the vast majority of cases.

Because of the increased incidence of infective endocarditis in patients with mitral valve prolapse, it is important to explain the risk to the patient. Most patients with significant prolapse will be prescribed antibiotics prior to certain dental or surgical procedures. When the condition is mild, however, antibiotics may not be needed.

In patients with chest pain or discomfort, certain drugs, such as propranolol (Inderal®) may improve the symptoms. When angina is suspected or cannot be ruled out, a stress test may be indicated. In patients with recurrent palpitations or dizziness and documented cardiac arrhythmias, antiarrhythmic drugs may be prescribed. In most cases, the arrhythmias are well tolerated and are not dangerous. Therefore, antiarrhythmic drugs are generally given only to alleviate bothersome symptoms and not to suppress the arrhythmia itself.

It should be emphasized, once again, that mitral valve prolapse is generally a benign condition, and that most patients will remain symptom-free for their entire lives and require, at most, reassurance and follow-up every year or so.

20 Congenital Heart Defects

A congenital heart defect is a malformation of the heart that is present at birth. It is estimated that approximately one percent of all infants are born with some type of congenital heart abnormality. The defect may be minor, requiring no treatment or restriction of activity; or, it may be so severe that no effective treatment is available and the infant will die. Between these two extremes, there is a wide range of congenital heart defects of various degrees of severity. When the problem is recognized early, many of these malformations can now be diagnosed accurately, and many of the babies can be saved with aggressive medical and surgical management.

Causes of Congenital Heart Defects

The development of the fetal heart is a very complex process during which a large number of malformations can occur. The human heart begins to develop from a single tube in about the third week of pregnancy, and starts beating at about the fourth week. The tube twists and divides in such a fashion as to form the four heart chambers, valves, and other structures. Congenital heart defects result from abnormal development of one or more structures in the fetal heart.

The cause for the malformation is only rarely identified. In fact, in over 95 percent of cases, the cause of the congenital defect will remain unknown even after a careful search for it. When a baby is born with a heart defect, the parents are often distressed and concerned about their own possible role in causing the problem. A specific cause, however, will be found in less than 5 percent of cases.

Some congenital heart defects can result from an infection, such as rubella (German measles), contracted by the mother during her pregnancy. Other times, disturbances in oxygen supply, deficiency of certain vitamins, or malnutrition of the pregnant mother may be associated with increased incidence of congenital abnormalities. Certain drugs and x-ray radiation, if received during the early months of pregnancy, can lead to cardiac defects in the developing fetus. Finally, several types of fetal chromosomal abnormalities, such as Down's syndrome (mongolism), are associated with an increased incidence of congenital heart defects.

The feasibility of prevention will depend upon what is learned in the future about the cause of the 90 percent or more of cardiac abnormalities for which no cause is found. An effective rubella vaccine has been developed, and immunization of children with this vaccine may eventually eradicate maternal rubella and its consequences.

No medications or drugs should be taken by the mother during her pregnancy without prior consultation with her physician. Similarly, the number of x-rays taken during pregnancy should be reduced to a minimum, in order to prevent irradiation of the developing fetus.

Common Congenital Defects

Normally, there is a continuous flow of blood throughout the circulatory system (see figure 10, page 65). The oxygen-poor blood coming from the entire body collects in the right atrium and then flows into the right ventricle. As the right ventricle contracts, it pumps blood into the pulmonary arteries and to the lungs. Within the lungs, carbon dioxide is released and fresh oxygen is picked up as we breathe. The oxygen-rich blood then flows into the left atrium and into the left ventricle (the main pumping chamber). As it contracts, the powerful left ventricle pumps blood under high pressure into the aorta (the body's main artery). The blood is then carried through large arteries, smaller arteries, and capillaries, and reaches the millions of cells in the different organs and tissues.

In the newborn baby (as well as in the adult), there exist two separate circulations: a) the *systemic circulation,* which carries oxygen-rich blood to the entire body, and which includes the left atrium, the left ventricle, the aorta, and the peripheral arteries; and b) the *pulmonary circulation,* which brings oxygen-poor blood back to the lungs, and which includes the right atrium, the right ventricle, and the pulmonary arteries.

The most common type of congenital heart defect results from the rerouting of blood flow within the heart and major blood vessels. Normally, the two circulations are separated from each other, and there is no direct communication between them. A shunt is the diversion of blood flow from one circulation to the other, due to the presence of a defect (hole). When a shunt is present, blood generally flows from the high-pressure systemic circulation to the low-pressure pulmonary circulation. This type of shunt is termed a "left-to-right shunt," because blood flows from the left side of the heart toward the right side of the heart.

Another common type of congenital heart defect results from obstruction to blood flow, either within the heart or in a major blood vessel near the heart. The obstruction is most frequently due to an abnormal narrowing (stenosis) of a heart valve. In some cases, the narrowing involves the aorta (the body's main artery). The presence of a narrowing anywhere in the circulation leads to a delay in the forward flow of blood, and thus results in backup of blood and increased pressures in the heart chambers located upstream to the narrowed area.

The seven most common cardiac defects (comprising over 80% of cardiac malformations present at birth) can be classified into three major groups, based on the primary congenital abnormality:

• An abnormal opening within the heart (or near the heart), resulting in a shunt (diversion of blood flow) between the systemic and pulmonary circulations.

• An abnormal narrowing at the level of the heart valves or the aorta, causing an obstruction to forward blood flow.

• A complex malformation (Tetralogy of Fallot), combining an abnormal shunt plus an obstruction to blood flow.

a) *Cardiac Defects Due to a Shunt*

There exists an abnormal opening (actually a hole) within the heart or near the heart. In general, the defect is found in one of three locations: it can be located in the wall separating the two atria (atrial septal defect); in the wall separating the two ventricles (ventricular septal defect); or at the level of the duct between the aorta and pulmonary artery (patent ductus arteriosus). The defect creates a shunt (diversion) from one circulation to the other. Blood generally flows from the high-pressure systemic circulation toward the low-pressure pulmonary circulation, creating a left-to-right shunt. Blood is "shunted" into the pulmonary circulation, thus increasing the volume of blood flowing through the lungs. (See figure 53).

Atrial Septal Defect. The abnormal opening is located in the atrial septum (the thin wall separating the left and right atria). Since the pressure is ordinarily greater on the left side of the heart, some of the oxygen-rich blood in the left atrium is forced through the defect, and gets mixed with the oxygen-poor blood present in the right atrium. From the right atrium, blood is forced into the right ventricle, and then pumped toward the lungs. As a result of the shunt, there is an increased volume of blood circulating within the right chambers of the heart, causing overloading of the right ventricle and increased blood flow through the lungs.

Ventricular Septal Defect. The defect is located in the ventricular septum (the muscular wall separating the two ventricles), thus creating an abnormal communication between the ventricles. Normally, during the contraction of the left ventricle (in systole) blood is pumped under high pressure into the aorta. When a ventricular septal defect is present, blood "leaks" through the hole, from the high pressure left ventricle toward the right ventricle, creating a left-to-right shunt. The left ventricle has to work harder in order to maintain normal cardiac performance, and the result is a progressive dilatation (enlargement) of the overworked ventricle.

Patent Ductus Arteriosus. In the unborn baby there is normally a special blood vessel, called ductus arteriosus, which connects between the pulmonary artery and the aorta. At birth, when the baby starts breathing on his own, the ductus normally closes off itself. In some babies, the ductus fails to close, and remains patent (open). This is particularly common in premature babies, who lack the normal mechanisms for duct closure because of immaturity. As a result of the opening, blood is diverted from the aorta into the pulmonary circulation, creating a left-to-right shunt. When the shunt is significant, a large volume of blood may be diverted through the ductus, and thus the left ventricle has to pump harder in order to maintain a satisfactory cardiac function.

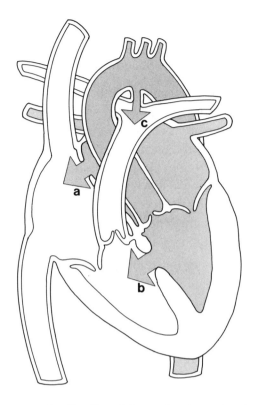

a - Atrial septal defect

b - Ventricular septal defect

c - Patent ductus arteriosus

Figure 53. Cardiac defects due to a shunt. There is diversion of blood from the high-pressure systemic circulation toward the low-pressure pulmonary circulation, creating a left-to-right shunt.

When the defect (either atrial septal defect, ventricular septal defect, or patent ductus arteriosus) is small, the overload is usually well tolerated. In patients with a large defect or long-standing disease, however, the pulmonary circulation may not be able to handle the large volume of blood. As a result, there may be a gradual alteration of the structure of the pulmonary blood vessels, which eventually begin to resemble arteries in the systemic circulation. These changes lead to increased resistance to blood flow, and therefore to increased pressures in the pulmonary circulation.

If the condition is not treated early enough, it may result in a severe and irreversible elevation of the pressures within the pulmonary circulation (a condition called pulmonary hypertension). When the pressure in the pulmonary circulation becomes higher than the pressure in the systemic circulation, oxygen-poor blood flows from the pulmonary circulation directly into the systemic circulation, thus creating a "reversal" of the shunt, which now becomes a right-to-left shunt.

b) Cardiac Defects Due to Obstruction to Blood Flow

The presence of a narrowing (stenosis) anywhere in the circulation leads to a delay in forward blood flow across the narrowed area. (See figure 54). This results in backup of blood and increased pressure in the heart chambers and blood vessels located upstream to the narrowed area. When a chronic pressure load exists, the body provides some relief in the form of compensatory mechanisms. There is usually thickening (hypertrophy) of the heart muscle, thereby strengthening the force of ventricular contraction. Over a period of years, the compensatory mechanisms eventually fail, and symptoms of heart failure develop.

Congenital Aortic Stenosis. In most cases, the narrowing is located at the level of the valve itself. There is usually fusion of the aortic cusps along their natural lines of closure (commissures), as well as thickening of the valvular tissue. Other times, the malformed valve has only two cusps instead of the normal three ("bicuspid" aortic valve). In most cases, the stenosis at birth is mild and the restriction to blood flow of little significance. Over the years, however, the thickened valve tends to thicken further, and there is also progressive calcification (deposits of calcium) of the cusps, leading to additional narrowing of the orifice.

When the narrowing of the aortic valve is significant, it results in slowing of blood flow across the valve during ventricular contraction (systole). In order to eject sufficient blood across the narrowed valve, the left ventricle has to generate higher pressures. The chronic pressure load leads to ventricular hypertrophy, that is, thickening of the ventricular heart muscle. Over the years, the stenosis becomes tighter, and the left ventricle may not be able to handle the increasing pressure load. The result is backing up of blood upstream to the failing ventricle, eventually leading to pulmonary congestion and symptoms of congestive heart failure.

Pulmonic Stenosis. The narrowing of the pulmonic valve is generally caused by the fusion of the valve cusps. Sometimes, it may be due to a buildup of extra fibrous tissue just above or just below the valve. In either case, the result is slowing of blood flow across the valve during the ejection period of the ventricle (systole). The right ventricle has to develop higher pressures in order to overcome the obstruction, and the compensatory mechanism for such a pressure burden is gradual hypertrophy (thickening) of the right ventricle.

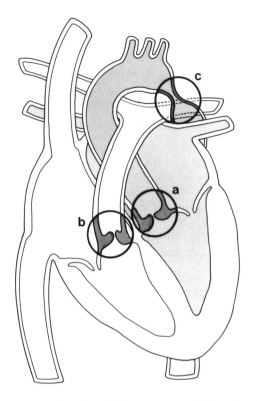

a - Aortic stenosis

b - Pulmonic stenosis

c - Coarctation of aorta

Figure 54. Cardiac defects due to obstruction to blood flow. An abnormal narrowing exists at the level of the heart valves or the aorta, causing a delay in forward blood flow.

In most patients with pulmonic stenosis, the right ventricle is able to handle the pressure load for a while. Over the years, however, the stenosis becomes tighter and the right ventricle may start failing. This leads to backup of blood upstream to the right ventricle, that is, in the peripheral veins, in the body organs, and in the lower extremities. Patients with severe or long-standing pulmonic stenosis eventually develop manifestations of "right-sided" heart failure, such as fatigue, congestion of the liver, and swelling of the legs (edema). At the same time there is often slowing of forward blood flow to the lungs. As a result, these patients often develop symptoms of fatigue and breathlessness on exertion.

Coarctation of the Aorta. The malformation consists of a significant narrowing (or constriction) of the aorta (the body's main artery). The narrowing is usually located at the level of the "aortic arch," just beyond the origin of the arteries conducting blood to the upper part of the body. The narrowing thus causes partial obstruction to the blood flowing through the aorta toward the lower part of the body. The result is an elevated blood pressure in the arms, neck and head, and a low blood pressure in the legs. As in aortic stenosis, the chronic pressure load eventually leads to hypertrophy of the left ventricle, the chamber located upstream to the narrowing. When the narrowing is severe or the condition long-standing, the left ventricle may fail, resulting in manifestations of heart failure.

c) A Complex Malformation: Tetralogy of Fallot

Tetralogy of Fallot is a complex malformation resulting from four different cardiac abnormalities, two of them major, and the other two of lesser importance. The two major abnormalities consist of:

a) A large defect (hole) between the two ventricles, creating diversion of blood flow (shunt) from one ventricle to the other.

b) A narrowing (stenosis) of the area beneath the pulmonic valve, causing obstruction to blood flow coming out of the right ventricle.

As we have seen, when an abnormal communication exists between the two circulations, blood generally flows from the high-pressure systemic circulation toward the low-pressure pulmonary circulation, creating a left-to-right shunt. In tetralogy of Fallot, however, things are different: the obstruction to blood flow creates a significant elevation of the pressure in the right ventricle, which may exceed the pressure in the left ventricle. As a result, a large volume of poorly oxygenated blood is diverted across the defect, from the high-pressure right ventricle into the left ventricle, creating a right-to-left shunt. (See figure 55).

If the obstruction to right ventricular outflow is severe, a large amount of poorly oxygenated blood may be diverted into the systemic circulation (hence into the general circulation), without first passing through the lungs. When the amount of oxygen-poor blood in the systemic circulation becomes excessive, it results in a bluish discoloration of the skin, fingernails, and lips, a condition termed cyanosis (see below).

Most infants with tetralogy of Fallot develop cyanosis before the age of one year, and they are commonly referred to as "blue babies." Other times, symptoms of cyanosis and shortness of breath develop in older children, typically during exertion, when the flow of oxygen-poor blood into the systemic circulation is the largest.

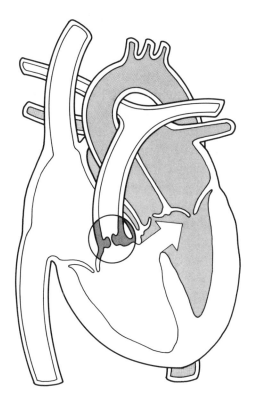

Figure 55. Tetralogy of Fallot. A complex malformation consisting of a large defect between the two ventricles and a narrowing of the pulmonic valve. Blood is diverted from the pulmonary circulation toward the systemic circulation, creating a right-to-left shunt.

Manifestations of Congenital Heart Disease

The clinical manifestations of congenital heart disease are variable, and depend on the type of defect and its severity. When the defect is small, the person may have no symptoms at all, and the problem is often discovered during a routine examination. When the defect is large, symptoms usually develop during childhood or adolescence. Finally, when the defect is severe, manifestations often develop at birth or during infancy.

Clinical Manifestations in Infants

Significant cardiac defects in the infant generally lead to manifestations of congestive heart failure. Although the mechanisms of heart failure are the same for all ages, the manifestations in the newborn infant are different than those in the adult patient. Shortness of breath (dyspnea) and fatigue express themselves as a feeding problem in the infant. Common symptoms are feeding difficulties, and failure to thrive (failure to gain weight and grow). If the problem is not recognized and diagnosed early, heart failure may progress rapidly during the first hours and days of life. In the older child, manifestations of heart failure may include shortness of breath, impaired growth, and delayed onset of puberty. Mental development, however, is rarely affected.

Another typical manifestation of congenital heart disease in infants and older children is cyanosis — a bluish discoloration of the skin, fingernails, and lips. It is caused by an excessive amount of oxygen-poor blood in the systemic circulation. Cyanosis is commonly seen in patients with tetralogy of Fallot, when there is passage of poorly oxygenated blood into the systemic circulation. In older children, cyanosis is usually precipitated by exertion, and relieved by rest.

Symptoms in Adults

Until 20 to 30 years ago, the only patients to survive to adulthood were those with simple, uncomplicated cardiac defects. However, this is no longer the case. Today, as new surgical procedures are being developed for almost all types of congenital heart defects, the life expectancy of these patients is much improved. When the defect at birth is severe, the patient may not be able to reach adulthood unless surgery is performed. When the congenital defect is small, on the other hand, symptoms may appear for the first time years later, during adolescence or adulthood.

In the adult patient, congenital heart disease is generally manifested by symptoms of heart failure. When the cardiac defect results in an excessive work load on the left ventricle, the clinical picture is usually that of "left-sided heart failure," with progressive shortness of breath due to pulmonary congestion. Initially, the symptoms may be mild and may occur only during strenuous exertion, but progressively they become more severe and occur at lower levels of activity. When the defect results in excessive burden on the right ventricle, the predominant manifestations are usually those of "right-sided heart failure," with predominant swelling of the legs and feet (leg edema), and congestion of the liver.

Congenital heart disease can lead to a variety of other cardiac symptoms. Palpitations, for example, may occur as a result of cardiac arrhythmias (disturbances of the heart rhythm), which can be associated with almost any type of heart disease. Chest pain occurs occasionally, and is generally the result of inadequate blood supply to the thickened or dilated left ventricle (such as in aortic stenosis). Syncope (fainting spell) is occasionally seen in patients with a narrowed valve, especially aortic stenosis and pulmonic stenosis. Syncope generally occurs during exertion, when the sudden increase in oxygen demand cannot be met because of the narrowing. Finally, nonspecific symptoms of heart failure, such as fatigue and weakness, can be seen as with almost any type of cardiac defect.

Diagnosing Congenital Heart Disease

The presence of congenital heart defects is usually suspected in patients who develop various cardiac manifestations, such as feeding difficulties (in infants), shortness of breath, fatigue, or cyanosis. The physical examination can provide additional clues regarding the nature of the defect, and the presence or absence of associated heart failure. Diagnostic tests will help confirm the suspected defect and assess its severity.

Physical Examination

Using his stethoscope, the doctor will auscultate (listen) over several areas of the chest. The normal heart sounds ("lub, dub... lub, dub...") are produced by the sudden closure of the heart valves during the various phases of the cardiac cycle. Abnormal heart sounds (such as "gallop," "click," and "snap") generally represent either a defective heart valve or weakness of the heart pump.

Heart murmurs result from turbulence in the bloodstream, and may represent a defective valve or an abnormal communication (shunt) within the cardiovascular system. The characteristics of the murmur (such as its timing during the cardiac cycle, the location on the chest wall where it is best heard, or its pitch quality) provide the physician with information regarding the specific valve involved, the type of valvular defect, or the presence of a shunt.

As part of a general physical examination, the doctor will also search for signs of congestive heart failure. For example, he will auscultate the lungs with his stethoscope, listening to the breath sounds. In patients with heart failure the lungs become congested, and crackling sounds (rales) can be heard over the lower portion of the chest during breathing. He will then examine the abdomen, especially the liver, which may become congested and enlarged in case of severe heart failure. Finally, he will also inspect the lower extremities for the presence of swelling (edema), which is often (but not always) a manifestation of heart failure.

Diagnostic Tests

Patients suspected of having a congenital heart defect will require at least two basic tests: an electrocardiogram (ECG) and a chest x-ray. If further information is needed, an echocardiogram will be performed to better visualize the heart structures. In patients with a significant defect or progressive symptoms, a cardiac catheterization is often necessary, in order to confirm the diagnosis and to assess the severity of the problem.

The *electrocardiogram (ECG)* is helpful in detecting the presence of chamber enlargement or hypertrophy. It is also of value in the diagnosis of cardiac arrhythmias, which are commonly present in patients with congenital heart disease. The chest x-ray is especially useful in the evaluation of cardiac chamber dimensions. The enlargement of a particular chamber affects the contour of the cardiac "silhouette" in a characteristic manner, thus helping to identify the chamber involved. In patients with congestive heart failure, small white patchy areas often appear within the lung fields, indicating congestion of the lungs.

The *echocardiogram* is of great value in the diagnosis of congenital heart defects. This noninvasive test provides accurate information about the heart valves, the size and function of the heart chambers, and the thickness of the ventricular walls. By carefully studying the tracings and pictures, the physician is able to identify the anatomic relationships between the heart chambers and the major blood vessels. He is thus able to define the anatomy of the heart and detect major defects or malformations.

Using the above noninvasive techniques, it is possible to diagnose with a reasonable degree of accuracy the majority of congenital heart defects. Cardiac catheterization is often required, however, in order to confirm the presence of a suspected defect and to assess the severity of the condition. The procedure is carried out routinely in all patients in whom a cardiac operation is contemplated.

During *cardiac catheterization,* a thin flexible tube (catheter) is inserted into a peripheral vein or artery and then directed toward the heart. The test allows the physician to measure the pressures within the heart chambers and major blood vessels. In patients with a narrowed valve, it is possible to measure the "pressure gradient" across the valve (the difference of pressure on both sides of the valve), and thus estimate the severity of the narrowing. In patients with a large septal defect and significant left-to-right shunt, the measurement of pressures may reveal the presence of an abnormal elevation of the pressures within the pulmonary circulation.

In patients with a septal defect, the presence of a shunt can be documented by obtaining multiple samples of blood from inside the heart chambers. In patients with an atrial septal defect, for example, there is an abnormal mixing of well-oxygenated blood coming from the left atrium with poorly oxygenated blood present in the right atrium. As a result of the mixing, there is an abnormal "step-up" of the oxygen saturation in the right atrium. The magnitude of the shunt can be then estimated by comparing the oxygen saturations at different levels within the heart chambers.

By selectively injecting dye into the heart chambers or major blood vessels (a procedure termed an angiogram), the physician can detect the presence of an abnormal communication. When a shunt is present, dye can be seen flowing from the chamber with higher pressure to the chamber with lower pressure. In patients with a ventricular septal defect, for example, dye is injected into the cavity of the left ventricle (left ventricular angiogram); dye can be seen passing through the hole (defect) and into the right ventricle, thus confirming the presence of a shunt.

Management of Congenital Heart Disease

As we have seen, the clinical manifestations of congenital heart disease are quite variable, and depend to a large degree on the type of defect and its severity. Some congenital cardiac abnormalities are so mild that they are barely noticeable. Others may correct themselves with time. Still others are serious enough to be life threatening or to interfere with the normal growth and development of the child. Generally, the major decision to be made in patients with congenital heart defects is whether medical management or surgical intervention is the preferred course of action.

Medical Treatment

Patients with congenital heart defects are at an increased risk of developing infective endocarditis. (See Chapter 21). Endocarditis is more likely to occur following certain dental and surgical procedures, during which there is release of bacteria into the bloodstream. These bacteria have a tendency to settle at or near the defect and cause an infection. In order to prevent infective endocarditis, most patients with known cardiac defects will be given preventive antibiotics ("prophylaxis") prior to and following certain dental and surgical procedures.

Patients who have developed manifestations of heart failure will be advised to get adequate physical and emotional rest, and to adjust the degree of their physical activity to the severity of their symptoms. Excessive salt and water retention, which often occurs in these patients, can be controlled with a low-salt diet, or with the use of diuretic drugs. In selected patients, the cardiac function can be improved with the use of digitalis drugs. Although some symptomatic patients will improve with medical therapy, the presence of symptoms in patients with a congenital heart defect is often an indication for a cardiac operation.

Surgical Treatment

An important decision in the management of patients with congenital heart disease concerns the timing of surgery. Patients with a small defect and only minimal symptoms may live for years with little or no change in their condition. In fact, spontaneous closure of small septal defects will occur in a significant number of patients.

Patients with a large defect or significant symptoms, on the other hand, may develop irreversible damage to the heart or blood vessels. In patients with a large septal defect, for example, the increased blood flow to the lungs may result in a severe and irreversible elevation of the pressures within the pulmonary circulation, and a "reversal" of the shunt (see above). Surgery is generally contraindicated in these patients, because little benefit and high mortality rates can be expected from repair of the defect.

The decision regarding the timing of surgery is generally based on the findings during the cardiac catheterization and on the patient's age. A routine cardiac catheterization is performed in all patients who are potential candidates for surgery. The presence of either a large septal defect or a significant valvular narrowing is usually a sufficient indication for surgery, even if the child has only minimal symptoms. If the disorder is not severe enough to demand immediate surgery, the operation is preferably delayed until the age of five or six. This delay allows the heart and blood vessels to become large enough for the surgeon to repair easily.

In patients with a septal defect (atrial or ventricular), surgical repair is generally indicated when a significant left-to-right shunt is present (as determined during cardiac catheterization), even if symptoms are minimal. If surgery is delayed for too long, this may result in severe and irreversible elevation of the pressure in the pulmonary circulation. The operation is ideally performed in children between three and six years of age, when they are big enough to withstand the stress of surgery. During the operation, the defect is closed either with a suture (stitch) or with a patch of prosthetic (artificial) material. The results of surgery are generally excellent, and the surgical mortality is low.

Patent ductus arteriosus is common in premature babies, who lack the normal mechanisms for duct closure because of immaturity. In these babies, the ductus can be sometimes stimulated to close by the administration of certain drugs. When a patent ductus is found in the full-term baby, the symptoms are usually milder, and many of the babies will reach adulthood without developing significant symptoms. A relatively common and potentially serious complication, however, is the infection of the ductus (similar to infective endocarditis). For this reason, the mere presence of a patent ductus in older children or adults is usually considered a sufficient indication for an operation. The procedure, which consists of a simple ligation (with a suture) of the ductus, is associated with a relatively low risk and a very low mortality rate.

Most children with valvular stenosis do not experience significant symptoms, and they usually grow and develop normally. In many of these children, the heart murmur is detected during a routine examination. When symptoms (such as shortness of breath, fatigue, fainting spells) do finally develop, the course of the disease accelerates, and most patients will become seriously ill unless a cardiac operation is performed. In patients who have pliable and non-calcified valves, a simple repair of the narrowed valve (by commissurotomy) is the preferred surgical technique. In most adult patients, the defective valve is rigid and calcified, and replacement with an artificial valve is often necessary.

The majority of children with coarctation of the aorta do not experience significant symptoms. The major hazards to children and adolescents with coarctation result from the severe elevation of the blood pressure. Complications may include the development of intra-cerebral (inside the brain) bleeding and congestive heart failure. For this reason, surgery is usually recommended for all patients with coarctation, even if symptoms are mild. The treatment consists of surgical resection of the area of narrowing and then suture of the two segments of the aorta back together. In young children, it is preferable to delay the surgery until the age of five or six. This allows the blood vessel to become large enough for the surgeon to repair easily, and is still early enough to avoid the complications from long-standing high blood pressure.

Tetralogy of Fallot is a complex congenital malformation that may lead to serious complications (such as recurrent spells of severe cyanosis, infective endocarditis, formation of blood clots, and bleeding problems). Total surgical correction of the malformation is therefore advisable for almost all patients with tetralogy. Because of the increased surgical risks in small infants, total correction is preferably delayed until childhood. A partial correction is often performed early in infancy, in order to increase the blood flow to the lungs and relieve the poor oxygenation of blood. Total correction is then carried out later, at a lower risk, during childhood.

21 Other Forms of Heart Disease

As we have seen, the most common form of heart disease results from the progressive narrowing of the coronary arteries (coronary heart disease). Other common types of heart disease result from long-standing elevation of the blood pressure (hypertension), disturbances of the cardiac rhythm (cardiac arrhythmias), defective heart valves (valvular heart disease), and cardiac defects present at birth (congenital heart disease).

There are also less common forms of heart disease. These conditions may involve the heart muscle (cardiomyopathies), the outer surface of the heart (diseases of the pericardium), or the inner surface of the heart (infective endocarditis).

Cardiomyopathies

Cardiomyopathies are diseases that primarily involve the heart muscle (myocardium). They are unique in the fact that they are *not* the result of other underlying conditions which can also damage the heart muscle (such as coronary heart disease, hypertension, valvular heart disease, or congenital cardiac defects).

Cardiomyopathies are classified into two major categories, according to the predominant type of functional impairment present:

• Dilated cardiomyopathies, characterized by significant dilatation (enlargement) and weakening of the left ventricle.

• Hypertrophic cardiomyopathies, characterized by marked hypertrophy (thickening) of the left ventricular walls.

It is sometimes useful to classify the cardiomyopathies into "primary" and "secondary" forms. The primary (or idiopathic) cardiomyopathies are conditions of the heart muscle that cannot be attributed to a specific cause. Secondary cardiomyopathies, on the other hand, are conditions in which the cause of the heart muscle abnormality is known, and is part of a disease process (such as a toxic reaction, an infection, or a metabolic disorder) that affects other organs in the body.

Dilated Cardiomyopathy

Dilated cardiomyopathy is a serious condition characterized by a progressive dilatation (enlargement) and weakening of the left ventricle. (See figure 56). In the majority of cases, the specific underlying cause cannot be found, and the condition is termed "idiopathic." Many cases of cardiomyopathy represent the end-result of damage to the heart muscle produced by a variety of toxic and infectious agents.

Among the toxic agents, excessive consumption of alcohol is a relatively common cause of heart muscle damage. This condition, termed alcoholic cardiomyopathy, is most commonly seen in middle-aged males who have been heavy consumers of whiskey, wine, or beer, usually for more than 10 years. Unless these patients completely abstain from alcohol, there is usually progressive and irreversible damage to the heart muscle.

In patients with dilated cardiomyopathy the weakened left ventricle is unable to pump blood efficiently. This eventually leads to backup of blood in the lungs and to manifestations of congestive heart failure. Common symptoms may include shortness of breath, fatigue, and leg swelling (edema). Some patients may experience palpitations, recurrent dizziness, and fainting spells (syncope), often the result of cardiac arrhythmias.

In some of these patients, there is a tendency for blood clots to form in the dilated and sluggish ventricle. These clots can become dislodged and travel through the circulation (they are then called emboli), and may end up in a peripheral artery, eventually causing tissue damage (such as stroke, heart attack, or blockage of the circulation to the legs).

The echocardiogram is the most useful test for the diagnosis of cardiomyopathies. This noninvasive technique can visualize the heart muscle, and thus allows an accurate assessment of its thickness and contractility. In these patients, the ventricle is markedly enlarged, and the contractility of the ventricular wall is "sluggish" and weak.

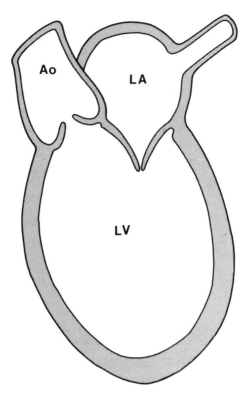

Figure 56. Dilated cardiomyopathy. The left ventricle (the main pumping chamber) is dilated and weakened.

Although a diagnosis of dilated cardiomyopathy can generally be made with noninvasive studies alone, invasive cardiac procedures (such as cardiac catheterization and coronary angiography) are often indicated. These tests are useful to confirm the diagnosis and to accurately assess the degree of ventricular weakening. The main purpose of these procedures, however, is to exclude the presence of surgically correctable abnormalities, such as heart valve defects or severe narrowing of the coronary arteries.

Since the underlying cause of dilated cardiomyopathy is generally unknown, specific treatment is not possible. Patients are advised to restrict their activities and adjust them according to the severity of their symptoms. Any strenuous activities must be avoided, since they may precipitate symptoms of heart failure. In patients with alcoholic cardiomyopathy, complete abstinence from alcohol is mandatory, in order to avoid continuing damage to the heart muscle.

Patients with dilated cardiomyopathy are generally not candidates for cardiac surgery, since the disease process involves the heart muscle itself. In symptomatic patients, treatment measures may include a low-salt diet, diuretics, digitalis drugs, and vasodilator drugs. Antiarrhythmic drugs may be used to treat cardiac arrhythmias. Patients with advanced disease are often treated with anticoagulant drugs ("blood thinners"), in order to prevent the formation of blood clots within the dilated ventricle.

Even with optimal therapy, the clinical course in patients with dilated cardiomyopathy is usually one of progressive deterioration, and the majority of patients will die within 4 to 5 years after the onset of symptoms. Rarely, cardiac transplantation may be an alternative. Considering the enormous emotional and economic investments required for carrying such a major surgery, however, this type of surgery is usually reserved only for carefully selected patients who are relatively young and active, and who do not have any other alternative for survival.

Hypertrophic Cardiomyopathy

Hypertrophic cardiomyopathy is characterized by marked thickening of the left ventricular walls. In one form of the disease (termed idiopathic hypertrophic subaortic stenosis, or IHSS) the septum (the muscular wall between the two ventricles) is markedly thickened, and as a result, there may be obstruction to the outflow of blood ejected from the left ventricle into the aorta. (See figure 57). The obstruction occurs when the mitral valve comes near and touches the thickened septum during the contraction of the ventricle (in systole).

In the majority of patients no specific cause for the disease can be found, so the condition is termed "idiopathic." In many cases the condition is inherited. In fact, about 50 percent of first-degree relatives (parents, siblings, children) will have some degree of thickening of the ventricular wall (on the echocardiogram), even though they may have no symptoms.

The symptoms of hypertrophic cardiomyopathy are variable. Some patients may never develop symptoms. The most common complaint in symptomatic patients is shortness of breath during exertion. Another common symptom is chest pain similar to angina, resulting from insufficient supply of blood to the markedly thickened heart muscle. Syncope (fainting spells) may occur during strenuous activity, resulting from the inability of the left ventricle to eject enough blood during exertion.

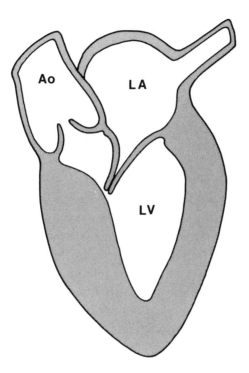

Figure 57. Hypertrophic cardiomyopathy. There is marked thickening of the left ventricular wall. There is also partial obstruction to blood flow, caused by the mitral valve nearly touching the septum during systole.

Cardiac arrhythmias are frequently seen in these patients, and may lead to significant symptoms such as palpitations, dizziness, and syncope. A rare but possible complication is sudden cardiac death. It is presumed to result from serious cardiac arrhythmias, but may also result from total obstruction to blood flow during strenuous activity.

The echocardiogram is by far the best technique for the diagnosis of hypertrophic cardiomyopathy. It reveals thickening of the ventricular wall, especially a disproportionate thickening of the septum. Cardiac catheterization may be performed in selected cases, to confirm the diagnosis, and to establish the presence or absence of obstruction to blood flow from the thickened septum.

Patients with hypertrophic cardiomyopathy are generally advised to avoid strenuous physical activity, because of the risk of severe and life-threatening symptoms. In symptomatic patients, the treatment of choice is with beta blockers or calcium channel blockers, which act by relieving, to some degree, the obstruction to blood flow.

If symptoms remain intractable despite optimal medical therapy, surgery may be considered in carefully selected patients. The surgical procedure consists of excision of a portion of the thickened septum, thus reducing the severity of obstruction to blood flow.

Diseases of the Pericardium

The pericardium is a thin fibrous membrane sac that surrounds the heart (see figure 58). It is composed of two layers of membrane separated by a film of lubricating fluid. The pericardium holds the heart in a fixed position, and enables the heart to move freely in relation to adjacent organs as it performs its pumping function. The two major conditions affecting the pericardium are the inflammation of the pericardium (pericarditis), and the presence of extra fluid within the pericardium (pericardial effusion).

Pericarditis

Pericarditis is due to inflammation of the pericardium. The inflammation causes roughening of the membrane surfaces, and may lead to the accumulation of fluid around the heart (pericardial effusion).

In the majority of cases, the specific cause of pericarditis is not known, and the condition is then termed "idiopathic" pericarditis. Known causes of pericarditis may include: viral infections, kidney failure, myocardial infarction, tuberculosis, malignancy, and auto-immune diseases (such as rheumatoid arthritis and systemic lupus erythematosus).

Pericarditis can also be seen in association with a number of conditions which have a common feature — a previous injury to the pericardium. For example, it may occur in patients who previously underwent a cardiac operation (during which the pericardium is dissected); or it may develop in patients who sustained a myocardial infarction (heart attack) a few weeks before. In either case, the mechanism involved is due to an auto-immune reaction that takes place during the healing process from the injury; the body erroneously develops antibodies against the injured tissue, and this may result in inflammation of the pericardium weeks or months later.

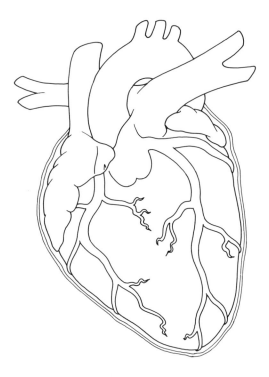

Figure 58. The pericardium is a thin fibrous membrane sac that surrounds and supports the heart.

Chest pain is by far the most common symptom seen in patients with pericarditis. The pain is often severe, localized to the middle of the chest, and often extending to the left shoulder. The pain generally lasts for hours, and may be mistaken for chest pain resulting from a myocardial infarction (heart attack). The pain is typically aggravated by taking a deep breath, coughing, swallowing, or turning in bed. It may be relieved by sitting up or leaning forward. A low-grade fever may be present, due to the presence of inflammation.

By applying a stethoscope to the chest area and listening carefully to the heart sounds, one may hear a characteristic squeaky, grating, high-pitched sound, called pericardial friction rub. It arises from the friction between the two inflamed layers of pericardium. This sound resembles the squeaky noise that results when rubbing two pieces of new leather together.

Typical ECG abnormalities usually occur a few hours or days after the onset of chest pain, evolving in a characteristic manner over the following few days. When there is a large amount of fluid around the heart (pericardial effusion), the chest x-ray may show an enlargement of the cardiac shadow. The echocardiogram is an excellent technique for the detection of smaller amounts of pericardial fluid.

The diagnosis of pericarditis is relatively simple, and is based on the clinical symptoms (chest pain), typical ECG abnormalities, and the presence of a small pericardial effusion on the echocardiogram. Most patients will require additional diagnostic tests in order to exclude the possibility of a more serious underlying condition, such as myocardial infarction, tuberculosis, malignancy, or auto-immune diseases. For this reason, most patients with pericarditis will be admitted to the hospital for observation and diagnostic work-up.

The treatment of pericarditis includes bed rest until pain and fever have disappeared. The chest pain usually responds to a variety of anti-inflammatory agents (such as aspirin). When the pain is severe and does not respond to these agents within a day or two, more potent anti-inflammatory drugs (such as corticosteroids), may be employed. Once the manifestations of pericarditis are under control, the next step is to establish whether or not the inflammation is related to another underlying condition (such as tuberculosis, rheumatoid arthritis, or malignancy) that may require further specific treatment.

Pericarditis is usually a self-limited condition, and the symptoms of inflammation gradually improve over a period of several days. The most troublesome complication, occurring in about one-fourth of patients, is the development of recurrent episodes at intervals of weeks or months after the initial episode.

A relatively rare complication is the development of a significant pericardial effusion which may interfere with the cardiac function (see below). For this reason, serial chest x-rays (or echocardiograms) are generally performed in patients recovering from an episode of pericarditis, in order to detect the build-up of fluid within the pericardium.

Rarely, there may be a slowly progressive scarring and thickening of the pericardium, over a period of years. Deposits of calcium may contribute to further stiffening of the pericardium. The persistent "constriction" of the heart by the stiffened pericardium may result in chronic constrictive pericarditis, a condition in which the ventricles are unable to fill up adequately with venous blood. Manifestations may include congestion of the liver, and swelling of the abdomen and legs. Chronic constrictive pericarditis is a progressive disease, and the only definitive treatment is a complete surgical resection ("strip-off") of the thickened pericardium.

Pericardial Effusion

Pericardial effusion is the abnormal presence of fluid around the heart, within the "pericardial sac" (see figure 59). Pericardial effusion generally develops as a response to inflammation of the pericardium. It may result from any of the conditions that can cause pericarditis (see above). When the cause of the pericardial effusion is unknown, it is termed "idiopathic."

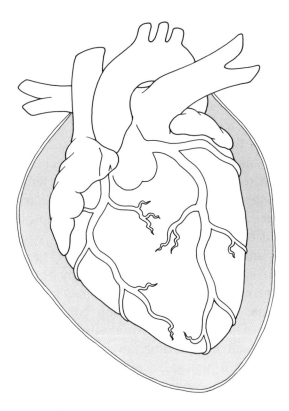

Figure 59. Pericardial effusion. A moderate amount of fluid is present around the heart, within the pericardial sac.

The effusion itself, even if large, generally does not cause any significant symptoms. When the effusion is associated with an inflammation of the pericardium (pericarditis), chest pain is usually present. A small or even a moderate pericardial effusion cannot be detected on physical examination alone.

The chest x-ray may show enlargement of the cardiac shadow when the effusion becomes moderate (over 10 oz., or 300 ml of fluid). When the effusion is large, the cardiac shadow often assumes a globular or "water bottle" shape. The echocardiogram is by far the most useful and accurate technique in the detection and assessment of the effusion. This sophisticated test is often able to detect as little as 1 oz. (30 ml) of fluid.

In most cases, pericardial effusion is well tolerated, and no specific treatment is required in patients with stable "idiopathic" pericardial effusion. Additional diagnostic tests are often necessary in order to detect or exclude the presence of an underlying condition (such as infection, tuberculosis, or malignancy).

In selected cases, a sample of the fluid is obtained during a procedure called pericardial tap (pericardiocentesis). A long needle is introduced by the cardiologist into the pericardium and a sample of fluid is aspirated with a large syringe. The characteristics of the fluid often provide clues regarding the nature of the underlying problem.

When the fluid in the pericardium accumulates slowly (that is, over a period of weeks or months), the pericardial sac stretches and may accommodate over a quart (or a liter) of fluid, without interfering with the heart function. On the other hand, when the fluid accumulates rapidly or when the effusion becomes very large, the result may be compression of the heart, a condition termed cardiac tamponade. The heart is unable to expand normally, and thus unable to fill up with blood during the relaxation period of the ventricles (in diastole). As a result, there may be a sudden decline of the cardiac function, eventually leading to the patient's death.

Cardiac tamponade is a life-threatening condition and therefore a medical emergency. Once the diagnosis is suspected on the basis of the clinical presentation, an echocardiogram is performed immediately to confirm the presence of a pericardial effusion. The treatment of cardiac tamponade is the immediate evacuation of the fluid with a pericardial tap. In some cases, the fluid may be drained with surgery, by performing a limited excision of the pericardium ("pericardial window").

Infective Endocarditis

The endocardium is the internal lining of the heart chambers, which includes the heart valves. Infective endocarditis, then, is the infection of the endocardium by bacteria (or other micro-organisms) which have entered the bloodstream. In most cases, the infection involves the heart valves, leaving the rest of the endocardium unaffected. Infective endocarditis is a very serious condition. When recognized early, it can be cured in most cases. However, if it is not diagnosed early enough and no treatment is given, the outlook is poor and the patient will probably die.

Although a large number of bacteria species can cause infective endocarditis, only a few account for the great majority of infections. The streptococci and staphylococci species, for example, cause more than 80 percent of all cases. Depending on the virulence of the bacteria, the clinical course of the disease can be slow and insidious ("subacute" endocarditis), or it can be rapid and abrupt ("acute" endocarditis).

Infective endocarditis occurs most commonly (but not always) in patients who already have a pre-existing abnormality of the heart valves, a congenital cardiac defect, or an artificial heart valve.

Under normal conditions, the heart tissue is not easily infected, and bacteria that may have entered the bloodstream are destroyed by the body's defense mechanisms (immune system). When the endocardium is already damaged or defective, however, bacteria circulating in the bloodstream may adhere to the abnormal roughened surface, where conditions are suitable for their growth. As the bacterial colony grows, it becomes covered by a clot, thus forming a barrier protecting the bacteria from the body's immune system. This explains why it may take a long time (several weeks or even months) to eradicate an established infection.

Most of the bacteria that cause infective endocarditis are normal inhabitants of the mouth, respiratory tract, gastro-intestinal tract, genito-urinary tract, and skin. The bacteria enter the bloodstream whenever there is disruption of the mucous membranes (the moist skin linings of the mouth and other internal organs) or the skin.

The entry of bacteria into the bloodstream most frequently occurs during dental procedures, and during various endoscopic manipulations (which involve the insertion of a tube into the body) or surgical procedures. The

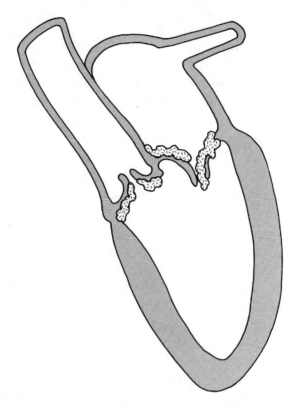

Figure 60. Infective endocarditis. Bacterial vegetations form on the heart valves, often causing interference with valvular function.

presence of bacteria in the blood also occurs frequently in drug addicts, who seldom use sterile techniques when injecting drugs into their veins.

The essential event leading to development of infective endocarditis is the attachment of bacteria circulating in the bloodstream onto the surface of the endocardium. Once lodged on the endocardium, the bacteria multiply and form bacterial colonies. Soon, there is formation of tiny blood clots, made of platelets (tiny blood cells) and fibrin material (a type of protein), which are then deposited around the growing bacteria.

As the bacterial colonies continue to grow, new layers of fibrin are deposited, resulting in the formation of bacterial vegetations (see figure 60), characteristic cauliflower-like and friable (easily crumbled) growths. The vegetations, which vary greatly in size, are usually located on the heart valves, and may lead to interference with the valvular function. In some cases, the vegetation can even destroy part of the valvular tissue. This may result in improper closure and leakage of the valve. There is also tendency for the friable vegetation to break off intermittently, sending small pieces (termed emboli) to various organs and sites in the body.

Clinical Manifestations

Symptoms of subacute endocarditis generally develop slowly and insidiously, over a period of several weeks or months. The patient usually develops recurrent fevers, which are often associated with chills and night sweats. Other nonspecific symptoms may include fatigue, weight loss, and joint pains. Symptoms generally persist and worsen over a period of several weeks before a diagnosis is made. The subacute form of endocarditis is particularly common in patients in whom a pre-existing defective valve is infected by bacteria of low-grade virulence.

In acute endocarditis, symptoms develop more rapidly, over a period of several days, and are usually more severe. Patients experience high-grade fever, shaking chills, and become very ill within a few days. The acute form is generally the result of an infection by a virulent type of bacteria, and may occur even in patients with perfectly normal heart valves. It is most frequently encountered in drug addicts who use intravenous drugs, and in the course of "blood poisoning" from serious infections.

As we just saw, bacterial vegetations may damage the valvular tissue or may interfere with the proper function of the valves. This may lead to impairment of the pumping function of the heart and may eventually result in manifestations of congestive heart failure. The nature of symptoms and their severity depends on the specific valve involved and the extent of the valvular damage or dysfunction. Depending on the severity of the damage, symptoms may progress over a period of months, weeks, or days.

Bacterial vegetations are often friable, and they can break off, sending small pieces of material (called emboli) into the bloodstream. This relatively common complication is termed embolization. Small emboli often go undetected, but large ones can cause obstruction to arteries, and may eventually result in tissue damage. For example, emboli can travel to the brain (causing a stroke), to the lungs (pulmonary emboli), to the coronary arteries (leading to a myocardial infarction), or to other vital organs such as the kidneys, bowel, and spleen.

Diagnosing Infective Endocarditis

The diagnosis of infective endocarditis is generally first suspected in patients with recurrent fever and a heart murmur. The fever is due to the presence of a bacterial infection. The heart murmur results from leakage of the infected valve. In patients with pre-existing valvular disease, the old murmur usually intensifies following the episode of endocarditis. Once the presence of infective endocarditis is suspected, further studies are necessary to confirm the diagnosis.

The echocardiogram is a very useful tool for the diagnosis of infective endocarditis. It is in fact the only test that can actually visualize the vegetations. It may show dense, fuzzy echoes attached to a heart valve, moving back-and-forth with the blood flow during the cardiac cycle.

An important step in the diagnosis of endocarditis is the isolation of the bacteria from the blood. It has been shown that almost all patients with infective endocarditis have a continuous presence of bacteria in the blood. The bacteria can be isolated by drawing blood cultures; several samples of blood are obtained, and then introduced into special culture bottles and left in an incubator for a period of a few days. If bacteria are present in the blood, they will continue to grow on the culture media, and the blood culture is then considered "positive." Once isolated, the bacteria can be identified, and the appropriate antibiotics can be given.

Treating Infective Endocarditis

Infective endocarditis is a very serious disease, and is almost always fatal unless treated. The principal goal of treatment is to kill and eradicate the invading micro-organisms. The optimal treatment is assured when treatment is begun early, when appropriate and effective antibiotics are selected, and when treatment is continued long enough to ensure that a relapse will not occur.

The appropriate antibiotics are selected according to the results of the blood cultures. In each case, the most potent available antibiotics are chosen, in order to assure eradication of the bacteria within the shortest time possible. When infective endocarditis is strongly suspected but results of blood cultures are not yet available, the patient is usually given a combination of several antibiotics. Treatment can be then adjusted several days later, when the specific organism is isolated and identified.

Bacterial colonies growing inside a vegetation are relatively well protected from the effects of the antibiotics. Therefore, patients with infective endocarditis usually require antibiotic therapy for a prolonged period of time (an average of 4 weeks), in order to achieve total eradication of the bacteria. Most patients will be hospitalized, at least initially, since the antibiotic drugs must be given by either intravenous or intramuscular injections. In order to achieve maximum effect, treatment regimens often combine two or more antibiotics.

In some cases of severe infective endocarditis, a cardiac operation may be indicated. The need for surgery most often arises in patients who suddenly develop manifestations of congestive heart failure as a result of a worsening valvular damage. Surgery may also be necessary in patients with one or more major episodes of emboli, in order to prevent their recurrence. Finally, an operation may be indicated in some patients who remain "septic" (infected) despite optimal antibiotic treatment.

The type of surgery most frequently performed is the replacement of the infected valve with an artificial valve. Correct timing of surgery is of critical importance. If the operation is undertaken too soon, the new valve can get infected by the same invading bacteria. If surgery is delayed for too long, on the other hand, the patient may suffer serious complications, such as severe heart failure or a stroke.

Preventing Infective Endocarditis

Dissemination of bacteria into the bloodstream often (but not always) occurs following certain dental and surgical procedures. The bacteria attach to the defective valve and eventually lead to infective endocarditis. A preventive antibiotic regimen, termed prophylaxis, is therefore routinely administered to susceptible patients with known heart defects, prior to certain dental and surgical procedures.

In general, individuals who are candidates for prophylaxis are those with valvular heart disease, congenital heart disease, or an artificial heart valve. Prophylaxis is generally indicated prior to dental procedures that are likely to result in gum bleeding (extraction of one or more teeth, cleaning and scaling of teeth). Prophylaxis is often recommended prior to surgery of the oral cavity (periodontal surgery), and upper respiratory tract (tonsillectomy); prior to various endoscopic procedures (such as bronchoscopy, upper GI endoscopy, and cystoscopy); prior to surgery of the respiratory, gastro-intestinal and genito-urinary tracts; and prior to drainage of abcesses or incision of infected tissues.

The regimen of antibiotics indicated for prophylaxis will vary according to the type of procedure being done. In a patient with valvular heart disease who undergoes a tooth extraction, for example, the physician may prescribe a dose of oral penicillin to be taken one hour prior to the procedure, and then several smaller doses to be taken over the following day or two. Some physicians may prefer, under certain circumstances, to administer the antibiotics by injection.

Despite the fact that prophylaxis is currently a widely used method, several uncertainties still exist regarding the specific indications for its use and the most effective antibiotic regimens. The American Heart Association has published recommendations for the use of prophylaxis in patients with underlying heart disease. Still, some physicians may have a different approach to the subject, and therefore each patient should consult his own physician regarding the need for antibiotics in specific circumstances.

Part Four

TREATING HEART DISEASE

22 Drugs for the Heart

A wide variety of drugs are now available for the treatment of patients with heart disease. Although quite effective, these drugs do not "cure" the disease. Rather, they are used to control and stabilize the abnormal condition (such as congestive heart failure, cardiac arrhythmias, or hypertension), and alleviate symptoms (such as chest pain, shortness of breath, or palpitations). Since most forms of heart disease have a chronic course, drug treatment generally becomes part of the patient's daily routine for periods of months and years.

These useful drugs have the potential of producing side effects and adverse reactions. There is probably no such thing as an effective cardiovascular drug that is perfectly safe. In fact, some mild side effects are often unavoidable if adequate doses of a drug are given. When prescribing a heart medication, the physician must therefore weigh the potential benefits from the drug against its possible side effects and adverse reactions. The patient, on his part, should inform the physician about any significant side effects that may occur.

There is generally no clearly defined dosage for any particular drug. Each patient's body will absorb and eliminate the drug at its own rate, and each patient will have a particular level of sensitivity to the drug. Because of these individual responses, what may be an effective dose for one patient may be a toxic dose for another patient. The role of the physician is to find the right drug and the correct dosage for the particular condition and the individual patient. This is done by increasing or decreasing the dosage until a point is reached where the drug can control the condition without resulting in significant side effects.

General Guidelines for Patients on Drug Therapy

• Since most types of heart disease have a chronic course, many of the cardiovascular drugs need to be taken on a regular basis over a period of months and years. Therefore, keep taking your pills even if you feel perfectly well, particularly if you feel perfectly well!

• The use of cardiovascular drugs is frequently associated with side effects and adverse reactions. Many side effects are mild and well tolerated by most patients. Others are bothersome and may even be dangerous. If you think you are experiencing a side effect, don't just stop treatment. Call your doctor and discuss the problem with him. Changes in your therapy can generally be made to overcome bothersome side effects.

• A wide variety of drugs are available for the treatment of heart disease. Different drugs are taken according to different schedules (some are taken once a day, others as often as four times a day). Therefore, be sure you understand the doctor's directions about the type of medications (for angina? heart failure? hypertension?), the times of the day to take them, and the precautions about anticipated side effects.

• Take your medications as directed. In order to remember, try taking your pills routinely at the same time of day. It's so easy to forget to take them, particularly when you feel well.

• If you miss a dose or two, don't take all the doses you have missed at one time, to "make up for the loss." Just get back on the prescribed schedule.

• Don't take other medications (including over-the-counter preparations) without telling your doctor. Certain medications may interact with each other, leading to reduced efficacy of the treatment, or bringing on other side effects.

• Stopping certain cardiovascular drugs abruptly may be dangerous. Therefore, never stop a medication without first consulting with your physician. Feeling better is never an excuse to reduce the dosage or to discontinue your medication abruptly.

A particular drug can be identified by its generic name, that is, its chemical name (verapamil, for example, is the generic name of one of the calcium channel blockers). The same drug can be also identified by its brand name, the name given by a particular drug company to identify its product (Calan® and Isoptin®, for example, are two brand names for verapamil, manufactured by two different pharmaceutical companies). In this book, brand names are shown with the sign ®. The price of a particular drug is generally higher (sometimes much higher) when it is sold under its brand name. By prescribing the brand name, however, the physician can be certain that his patient will receive a preparation of the best quality.

Cardiovascular drugs are classified according to the condition for which they are most often prescribed (antianginals, antiarrhythmics, antihypertensives, etc.). They can also be classified in groups, according to their predominant mechanism of action (beta blockers, calcium channel blockers, diuretics, etc.). A particular drug can be used in the treatment of several different conditions. Beta blockers, for example, are effective agents used in the treatment of angina, cardiac arrhythmias, and hypertension.

The following pages offer a brief description of some of the most commonly prescribed cardiovascular drugs, grouped according to their predominant mechanism of action, and listed alphabetically by brand name. Only the most common side effects or the most important ones (although their incidence may be small) are listed.

Antianginal Drugs

Angina is a discomfort in the chest that results from myocardial ischemia ("starving" of the heart muscle for oxygen). Myocardial ischemia occurs whenever the available oxygen supply to the heart muscle does not meet the oxygen demand (see Chapter 13). Treatment of angina, therefore, is aimed at either reducing the oxygen requirements of the heart muscle, or increasing the coronary blood flow. Antianginal drugs favorably affect the imbalance between myocardial oxygen demand and supply, and are therefore capable of relieving or preventing angina attacks. The three major classes of antianginal agents available are the nitrates, the beta blockers, and the calcium channel blockers.

a) *Nitrates*

Tablets:
- Cardilate® (erythrityl tetranitrate)
- Isordil® (isosorbide dinitrate)
- Nitro-Bid® (nitroglycerin)
- Nitrostat® (nitroglycerin)
- Peritrate® (pentaerythritol tetranitrate)
- Sorbitrate® (isosorbide dinitrate)

Skin patches:
- Nitro-Dur® (nitroglycerin)
- Nitrodisc® (nitroglycerin)
- Transderm-Nitro® (nitroglycerin)

Ointment:
- Nitrol® (nitroglycerin)

Actions: The nitrates are primarily vasodilator drugs; they relax the walls of blood vessels (both veins and arteries), thus causing them to dilate. As a result of these actions, the heart has less work to perform and therefore needs less oxygen. On the supply side, nitrates increase blood flow to the heart muscle by relaxing the walls of the coronary arteries and by relieving coronary spasm.

Indications: Nitroglycerin remains the most effective drug for the relief of an angina attack. During an episode of angina, a tiny nitroglycerin tablet is placed under the tongue and allowed to dissolve, often producing a slight tingling sensation. The angina pain is usually relieved within a few minutes. In addition to the rapid-acting nitroglycerin preparations, there are several long-acting nitrates, used for the prevention of angina attacks. These preparations are ineffective in relieving angina once it has occurred, but are useful in preventing the onset of symptoms. They are administered one to several times a day depending upon their duration of action.

Nitrate preparations: The oral preparations (tablets and capsules) are taken 3 or 4 times a day. The nitroglycerin ointment is applied to the skin (most commonly the chest) 3 or 4 times a day. More recently, transdermal patches have made the delivery of nitroglycerin more convenient and less messy.

The patch is applied to the skin once a day, and nitroglycerin gradually diffuses through the skin at a constant rate, over a period of 24 hours.

Possible side effects: Nitrates are generally safe and well tolerated. The most common troubling side effect, seen in approximately 25% of patients, is headache. It is often possible to eliminate or minimize the headache by starting with small dosages and slowly working up to effective dosages, or simply by taking a pain-killer to relieve the headache. Another relatively common side effect is postural hypotension, that is, the sudden onset of dizziness or faintness upon standing. If an episode of postural hypotension occurs, the patient should sit or lie down immediately until symptoms have improved, and then should notify his physician. Other side effects that may occur with the use of nitrates are flushing, dizziness, palpitations, weakness, stomach upset, and skin rash.

b) Beta Blockers

- Blocadren® (timolol)
- Corgard® (nadolol)
- Inderal® (propranolol)
- Lopressor® (metoprolol)
- Normodyne® (labetalol)
- Tenormin® (atenolol)
- Trandate® (labetalol)
- Visken® (pindolol)

Actions: The beta blockers act primarily on the heart. They block the action of the beta receptors, that is, the nerve endings that affect the heart rate and force of contraction. The result is a slowing of the heartbeat, as well as a decrease of the force of cardiac contraction. By their action, they reduce the amount of work performed by the heart, and therefore reduce myocardial oxygen demand.

Indications: The beta blockers are effective agents for the treatment and prevention of angina. Beta blockers are sometimes prescribed to patients recovering from a heart attack (studies have shown that the use of beta blockers in such patients can help reduce the risk of sudden death and recurrent heart attack). The beta blockers are also used for the treatment of hypertension and for the control of certain cardiac arrhythmias.

Possible side effects: The beta blockers are generally well tolerated, but nevertheless, certain adverse reactions can result from their use. When given to patients with severely weakened heart function, they may bring on symptoms of heart failure. In patients with chronic lung disease or asthma, they may cause worsening of shortness of breath and wheezing. Some slowing of the heart rate is to be expected in most patients. If an overly large dose is taken, however, they may cause excessive slowing of the heartbeat, occasionally resulting in symptoms of dizziness. Other possible side effects include tingling of the extremities (hands and feet), cold extremities, stomach upset, fatigue, mental depression, and skin rash.

Precautions: There have been reports of worsening angina, heart attacks, and even sudden death, following abrupt stopping of beta blockers in patients on long-term treatment. For this reason, patients should never stop taking beta blockers abruptly and without their physician's knowledge.

c) Calcium Channel Blockers

- Calan® (verapamil)
- Cardizem® (diltiazem)
- Isoptin® (verapamil)
- Procardia® (nifedipine)

Actions: These agents block calcium transport mechanisms in blood vessels and heart muscle cells (which require the presence of calcium ions in order to contract). Calcium channel blockers relax the walls of the coronary arteries, and thus prevent coronary spasm (the temporary contraction of a segment of the arterial wall). In addition, they act directly on the heart muscle cells, causing a slight decrease in contractility, therefore reducing myocardial oxygen demand.

Indications: Because of their ability to relax the coronary arteries, calcium channel blockers are effective in the treatment of coronary spasm. They are also effective in the treatment and prevention of angina, especially in patients who continue having symptoms despite optimal doses of nitrates and beta blockers.

Possible side effects: The calcium channel blockers differ in the type and incidence of reported side effects. Nifedipine, for example, is more likely to produce hypotension (low blood pressure). Verapamil and diltiazem, on the other hand, are more likely to interfere with the cardiac conduction system and thus result in excessive slowing of the heartbeat. Because of their direct action on the heart muscle, any of the calcium channel blockers may cause worsening of heart failure. Other possible side effects include: leg swelling (mostly nifedipine), constipation (verapamil), headache, dizziness, palpitations, fatigue, stomach upset, and skin rash.

Diuretics

Thiazide diuretics:
- Enduron® (methychlothiazide)
- Esidrix® (hydrochlorothiazide)
- HydroDiuril® (hydrochlorothiazide)
- Hygroton® (chlorthalidone)
- Zaroxolyn® (metolazone)

"Loop" diuretics:
- Bumex® (Bumetanide)
- Lasix® (furosemide)

Potassium-sparing agents:
- Aldactone® (spironolactone)
- Dyrenium® (triamterene)
- Midamor® (amiloride)

Diuretic combinations:
- Aldactazide® (spironolactone & thiazide)
- Dyazide® (triamterene & thiazide)
- Maxzide® (triamterene & thiazide)
- Moduretic® (amiloride & thiazide)

Actions: The diuretics act primarily by increasing the excretion of salt and water into the urine, leading to reduction of the amount of fluid in the circulation and therefore lowering of the blood pressure. The most commonly employed diuretics are the thiazides (used primarily in the treatment of hypertension), and the more potent "loop" diuretics (used primarily in the treatment of heart failure).

Indications: The diuretics are effective in the management of congestive heart failure. They lessen fluid retention and edema, and lead to improvement in shortness of breath. Diuretics are also used in the treatment of hypertension. Many physicians use a diuretic as the first-step drug in the initial treatment of mild hypertension. A diuretic can also be added to other antihypertensive drugs when a combination of several medications is needed to control the blood pressure.

Possible side effects: The diuretics are generally well tolerated. Their use, however, can be associated with a number of side effects, some of them potentially serious. Most diuretics cause loss ("wasting") of potassium into the urine, thus causing depletion of body potassium. A low potassium level can result in symptoms of weakness and fatigue, leg cramps, and palpitations; it can also lead to serious disturbances of the cardiac rhythm. Loss of potassium can be counteracted by eating potassium-rich foods (such as fruits and vegetables), or by taking potassium supplements or potassium-sparing agents (see below). Other side effects associated with the use of diuretics include: postural hypotension, dizziness, headache, stomach upset, and skin rash.

Potassium supplements: These preparations contain potassium chloride, and are available as liquid, tablets, or capsules. Some of the common preparations are: Kaochlor®, Kaon®, Kay Ciel®, K-Lor®, Klorvess®, Klotrix®, K-Lyte®, K-Tab®, Micro-K®, and Slow-K®. Side effects associated with these preparations may include abdominal discomfort, intestinal irritation, and diarrhea.

Potassium-sparing agents: These are weak diuretics that prevent the depletion of potassium induced by the thiazide (or loop) diuretic. They are generally employed in combination with a thiazide diuretic ("diuretic combinations"), and are thus able to counteract the loss of potassium induced by the diuretic.

Precautions: Patients taking diuretics should eat foods rich in potassium (such as bananas, oranges, tomatoes) in order to avoid excessive potassium loss. Many patients will eventually require the addition of potassium supplements or potassium-sparing agents.

Important: Patients taking a potassium-sparing agent (or a diuretic combination) should not take extra potassium supplements (unless directed by a physician), since this may lead to a dangerous rise in the potassium blood level.

Cardiac Stimulants: Digitalis

- Lanoxin® (digoxin)

Actions: Digitalis drugs increase the contractility (force of contraction) of the heart muscle, and thus improve the performance of the failing heart. As antiarrhythmic agents, they slow down the transmission of the atrial impulses through the AV node (the "gateway" to the ventricles), and thus slow down the rate at which the ventricles beat.

Indications: Digitalis drugs are used in the treatment of congestive heart failure, often in combination with diuretics. They are also effective in the management and prevention of certain cardiac arrhythmias.

Possible side effects: Digitalis drugs are quite effective, but they must be taken under close medical supervision, since they can result in potentially serious toxic reactions. Excessive amounts of the drug can accumulate in the body and may lead to digitalis toxicity. The most serious effects of digitalis toxicity are disturbances in the cardiac rhythm, which may be extremely serious. Other toxic manifestations are varied and often nonspecific, and may include: loss of appetite, nausea and vomiting, diarrhea, drowsiness, visual disturbances (blurred or colored vision), headache, dizziness, and fatigue.

Precautions: In most patients, the amount of digitalis needed to strengthen the heart is close to the amount that is likely to cause side effects and toxicity. Therefore, digitalis drugs must be taken only under close medical supervision. Patients must never take an extra dose of digoxin ("just to strengthen the heart"), unless directed by the physician. The physician should be notified without delay if any of the manifestations that suggest a possible toxicity have developed.

Antiarrhythmics

- Inderal® (propranolol)
- Lanoxin® (digoxin)
- Norpace® (disopyramide)
- Procan SR® (procainamide)
- Pronestyl® (procainamide)
- Quinaglute® (quinidine)
- Quinidex® (quinidine)
- Tambocor® (flecainide)
- Tonocard® (Tocainide)

Actions: Propranolol (a beta blocker) acts by blocking the action of adrenaline on the beta receptors in the heart; the result is a slowing of the heartbeat. Digoxin (a digitalis drug) slows down the transmission of atrial impulses through the AV node (the "gateway" to the ventricles), thus slowing down the rate at which the ventricles beat. Disopyramide, procainamide, quinidine, flecainide, and tocainide act primarily by suppressing the irritable discharging sites that are responsible for the arrhythmia.

Indications: Antiarrhythmic drugs are used in the treatment and prevention of cardiac arrhythmias. (See Chapter 17). A particular drug may be used for the treatment of more than one type of arrhythmia. Quinidine, for example, is used primarily in the treatment of ventricular arrhythmias, but is also effective in the treatment and prevention of certain atrial arrhythmias. There is generally more than one way to treat a specific arrhythmia, but there is usually one specific drug that is the most effective one for that particular situation (the "drug of choice").

Possible side effects: Side effects associated with the use of antiarrhythmic drugs vary widely depending on the particular drug used. Side effects commonly encountered with these drugs include: nausea, stomach upset, fatigue, dizziness, headache, palpitations, and skin rash. In excessive doses, most antiarrhythmic drugs will cause some degree of toxicity, especially on the cardiovascular system. Such toxic reactions may include hypotension (low blood pressure), worsening of heart failure, or the induction of serious cardiac arrhythmias (which may be even more dangerous than the original arrhythmias for which the drug was initially prescribed!).

Antihypertensives

Hypertension (high blood pressure) is a condition characterized by an excessive amount of pressure within the arteries. In general terms, hypertension may result either from an increase in the amount of blood pumped by the heart, or from constriction (tightening) of the peripheral arteries. The heart, kidneys, and autonomic nervous system all play an important role in the regulation and control of the blood pressure. The various antihypertensives act at different levels within this complex system. Five major classes of drugs, each with a different mechanism of action, are currently used in the treatment of hypertension. (See also Chapter 15). The two most commonly used classes of antihypertensive drugs, namely the diuretics and beta blockers, were already discussed above.

a) Diuretics

The diuretics ("water pills") act primarily by increasing the elimination of salt and water into the urine. Their action leads to reduction of the amount of fluid in the circulation and thus to lowering of the blood pressure. Most physicians still use a diuretic as the first-step drug in the initial treatment of hypertension. A diuretic is often added to other antihypertensive drugs when a combination of several medications is needed to control the blood pressure. The major side effect resulting from the use of diuretics is the loss ("wasting") of potassium in the urine, which may lead to symptoms of leg cramps, fatigue, and palpitations. (For further discussion on diuretics, see above, page 282).

b) Beta Blockers

The beta blockers act primarily by blocking the stimulation of the beta receptors, that is, the nerve endings that affect the heart rate and the force of contraction. By their action, they cause a decrease in the amount of blood pumped by the heart and thus lead to lowering of blood pressure. A beta blocker can be prescribed as a first-step drug in the initial treatment of hypertension, or it can be added as a second drug in patients who were previously treated with a diuretic alone. (For further discussion on beta blockers, see above, page 280).

c) *Centrally Acting Drugs*

- Aldomet® (methyldopa)
- Catapres® (clonidine)
- Ismelin® (guanethidine)
- Serpasil® (reserpine)
- Wytensin® (guanabenz)

Actions: These agents act by blocking the transmission of impulses within the autonomic nervous system (which controls the involuntary action of various internal organs, including the heart, lungs, and blood vessels). By their action, they induce dilatation of the peripheral arteries, and thus lower the blood pressure.

Indications: These drugs are usually reserved for patients with moderate or severe hypertension who have not responded to treatment with milder medications (such as diuretics and beta blockers).

Possible side effects: Their incidence varies among the various agents in this group. The most troublesome side effect is postural hypotension, that is, the sudden drop of blood pressure upon standing. This may lead to symptoms of lightheadedness and faintness. Other possible side effects include palpitations, nausea, stomach upset, dizziness, weakness, dry mouth, headache, drowsiness, sedation, depression, and impotence.

Precautions: If an episode of postural hypotension occurs (sudden onset of dizziness or faintness upon standing), the patient should sit or lie down until symptoms improve, and then should notify his physician.

d) *Vasodilators*

- Apresoline® (hydralazine)
- Loniten® (minoxidil)
- Minipress® (prazosin)

Actions: Vasodilators lower the blood pressure by relaxing the vascular smooth muscle of the peripheral arteries, causing them to dilate. As a result of vascular dilatation, the resistance to blood flow is reduced, and the blood pressure is lowered.

Indications: The vasodilators are potent drugs, and their use is generally reserved for patients with moderate or severe hypertension who have not responded to treatment with milder medications.

Possible side effects: The major drawback in the use of vasodilator drugs is their tendency to cause a reflex acceleration of the heart rate, as well as retention of salt and water. Other side effects may include postural hypotension, headache, dizziness, leg swelling, nausea, stomach upset, weakness, and depression.

Precautions: If an episode of postural hypotension occurs (sudden onset of dizziness or faintness upon standing), the patient should sit or lie down until symptoms improve, then should notify his physician.

e) *Angiotensin Inhibitors*

- Capoten® (captopril)

Actions: Angiotensin is a naturally occurring substance that induces an elevation of the blood pressure through two mechanisms: constriction (tightening) of the small peripheral arteries, and retention of salt and water. The angiotensin inhibitors lower the blood pressure by inhibiting (blocking) the actions of angiotensin.

Indications: The use of these agents is reserved for patients with moderate or severe hypertension, when other milder agents have not been effective in controlling the blood pressure.

Possible side effects: The use of angiotensin-inhibitor agents is associated with a relatively high incidence of serious adverse reactions, such as hypotension (low blood pressure), kidney problems, and abnormalities of the blood count. Other side effects may include rapid heartbeat, palpitations, dizziness, and skin rash.

f) *Combinations of Antihypertensives and Diuretics*

- Aldoril® (methyldopa & thiazide)
- Apresazide® (hydralazine & thiazide)
- Combipres® (clonidine & thiazide)
- Corzide® (nadolol & thiazide)

- Diupres® (reserpine & thiazide)
- Esimil® (guanethidine & thiazide)
- Inderide® (propranolol & thiazide)
- Minizide® (prazosin & thiazide)
- Tenorectic® (atenolol & thiazide)
- Timolide® (timolol & thiazide)

These combination drugs have fixed dosage levels, and therefore are generally not used for the initial treatment of hypertension (when frequent adjustments of dosages are necessary). Rather, they are useful when there is a need to add a second antihypertensive drug, therefore giving the convenience of taking only one pill instead of two.

Anticoagulants

- Coumadin® (warfarin)

Actions: Anticoagulants ("blood thinners") act by interfering with the production of several factors which are active in the blood coagulation (clotting) mechanism. By their action, they prevent the formation of blood clots within the circulatory system.

Indications: They are prescribed for the treatment and prevention of blood clot formation within the heart and blood vessels.

Possible side effects: The use of anticoagulants is associated with an increased risk of bleeding. Internal bleeding may be manifested by the presence of blood in the stools or urine. Other side effects may include skin rash, easy bruising of skin, nausea, diarrhea, and abdominal cramps.

Precautions: It is important to take anticoagulants exactly as prescribed by the doctor. Aspirin must not be taken with the anticoagulants (unless directed by the doctor), since this may result in an increased tendency for bleeding. Patients should take steps to avoid accidental cuts and scrapes as much as possible (for example, by using an electric razor or a soft toothbrush). It is important to notify the doctor of any unusual bleeding, such as blood in the stools (or black, tarry stools), blood in the urine, heavier than usual menstrual flow, or bruising of the skin.

Cholesterol-Lowering Drugs

- Colestid® (colestipol)
- Lorelco® (probucol)
- Nicolar® (niacin)
- Questran® (cholestyramine)

Actions: In general terms, cholesterol-lowering drugs act through two basic mechanisms: some of these agents prevent the absorption of dietary cholesterol from the gastro-intestinal tract; others simply reduce the synthesis of cholesterol in the liver. Through their actions, they lower the level of cholesterol in the blood.

Indications: Cholesterol-lowering drugs are indicated in patients with an excessive amount of cholesterol in the blood (hypercholesterolemia). They may also be prescribed to patients with an only moderate elevation of blood cholesterol, in order to reduce the risk of coronary heart disease. Although several large-scale studies have shown that lowering blood cholesterol in patients with mild to moderate hypercholesterolemia may reduce their risk of coronary heart disease, the actual level of cholesterol for which drug treatment should be initiated is still being debated.

Important: It must be emphasized that a prudent low-fat, low-cholesterol diet (see Chapter 4) is the first line of treatment in patients with an elevated blood cholesterol level. With the help of readily available teaching materials and nutrition counseling, most patients will be able to achieve a meaningful reduction in their blood cholesterol. In those individuals in whom adequate reductions cannot be achieved through dietary changes alone, cholesterol-lowering drugs can be helpful.

Possible side effects: In general, cholesterol-lowering drugs cause frequent side effects, usually mild but sometimes more serious. The various drugs differ in the type and incidence of reported side effects. The most common ones involve the gastro-intestinal tract, especially constipation, heartburn, nausea, bloating, abdominal cramps, and unpleasant taste. Other possible side effects include headache, dizziness, and palpitations; diarrhea (with probucol); and flushing of skin (with niacin).

Antiplatelet Drugs

- Bayer Aspirin® (aspirin)
- Bufferin® (aspirin)
- Ecotrin® (aspirin)
- Persantine® (dipyridamol)

The platelets are tiny blood cells that have an important function in the blood-clotting mechanism. When a blood vessel is injured, the platelets begin sticking to the vessel wall and to each other, thus forming a clot at the damaged site. The clot helps to patch the damaged wall and prevent further bleeding. In certain circumstances, the formation of blood clots may cause serious problems. In patients with coronary artery disease, for example, there is an increased tendency for blood clots to form at the site of the plaque; this, in turn, can lead to complete blockage of the coronary artery and result in a myocardial infarction (heart attack).

Actions: Antiplatelet drugs help keep the platelets from sticking to the blood-vessel walls and to each other; this way, they reduce the tendency for blood-clot formation.

Indications: Studies have shown that aspirin (and, to a lesser degree, dipyridamol) can help reduce the risk of a heart attack in patients who have already suffered a heart attack, and in patients with unstable angina. These products are also used in patients after coronary bypass surgery, to reduce the risk of closure of the bypass graft.

Possible side effects: The use of antiplatelet drugs is associated with a slight bleeding tendency. Other side effects include stomach upset, dizziness, allergic reactions, and skin rash.

23 Coronary Balloon Angioplasty

Coronary balloon angioplasty (also termed percutaneous transluminal coronary angioplasty, or PTCA) is a sophisticated technique used to dilate the coronary arteries at the point where they have become narrowed by a plaque. This relatively new procedure, first introduced in the late 1970s, has become an alternative to coronary bypass surgery in selected patients with coronary artery disease.

During the angioplasty procedure, a special catheter with a tiny balloon at its tip is passed through an artery in the leg (or arm) and guided into the diseased coronary artery. When the balloon reaches the narrowed portion of the artery, it is inflated, thus compressing the plaque against the arterial walls. When the catheter is withdrawn, the plaque remains compressed, therefore allowing a better flow of blood to the heart muscle.

Before the Procedure

Before an angioplasty can be considered, patients must first undergo cardiac catheterization and coronary angiography (see Chapter 10), in order to visualize the coronary arteries and assess the severity of the narrowings (called "lesions"). In general, the coronary angioplasty is performed a day or two after the coronary angiogram. Sometimes, the patient is sent home following the coronary angiogram, then re-admitted the day before the coronary angioplasty.

As with cardiac catheterization, several routine laboratory tests (such as ECG, chest x-ray, and blood tests) are performed prior to the procedure.

The physician who is to perform the angioplasty (a specially trained cardiologist) then explains the procedure to the patient, its potential benefits, as well as its possible risks. The patient is then asked to sign a consent form, thus giving the doctor permission to perform the procedure. As we will see, some patients undergoing angioplasty may develop major complications and require emergency bypass surgery. For this reason, patients are generally asked to sign a consent for a possible coronary bypass surgery as well.

If the angioplasty is scheduled for the next morning, no food or drink is allowed after midnight. If the procedure is scheduled for the next afternoon, however, a light breakfast may be permitted. As with catheterization, an area of the groin (or sometimes the arm) is cleansed and shaved. An intravenous line is inserted into a vein in the arm, and kept open by a slow infusion of sugar solution. Patients are usually given mild sedation before leaving their room, in order to alleviate apprehension and reduce anxiety.

During Coronary Angioplasty

Coronary balloon angioplasty is performed in the cardiac catheterization laboratory ("cath lab"). The equipment used for angioplasty is essentially similar to that used for catheterization, and includes a large x-ray camera, television screens, cardiac monitors, and other instruments and devices. As with catheterization, the patient is transported to the cath lab on a movable bed, and then transferred to the x-ray table. In order to prevent contamination during the procedure, the patient is draped with sterile sheets, and the staff wears sterile gowns, masks and gloves.

As with catheterization, the angioplasty procedure involves the insertion of a catheter into the groin area (or sometimes the arm). The site where the catheter will be inserted is cleansed thoroughly with an antiseptic solution, and a local anesthetic is injected into the skin with a small needle, to numb the area. This may cause a mild stinging sensation (like a "bee sting"). A tiny incision is made in the skin, and a large needle is used to puncture the artery. A soft and flexible metallic wire (guide wire) is inserted into the artery. A short hollow plastic tube, called an introducer sheath, is then slipped over the guide wire and into the artery. It is through this introducer sheath that the catheter will be inserted.

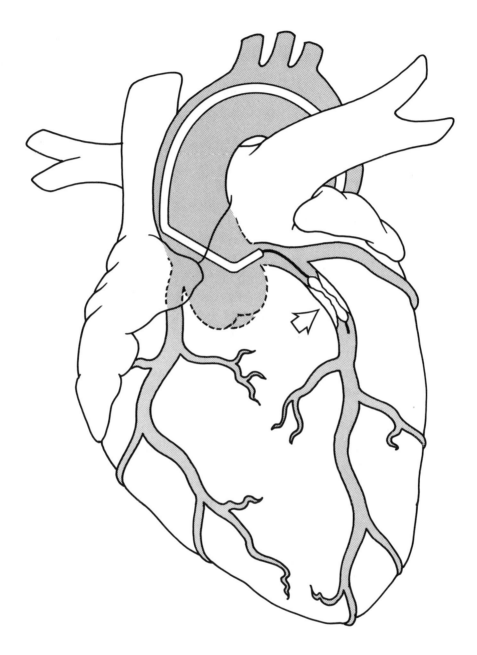

Figure 61. Coronary balloon angioplasty. The guiding catheter is directed toward the opening of the coronary artery. The thinner dilatation catheter is then threaded through the guiding catheter and advanced into the coronary artery, until the balloon reaches the area of narrowing.

Next, a relatively large size catheter, called a guiding catheter, is inserted through the introducer sheath, into the artery. It is called a "guiding" catheter because it acts as a guide for the thinner catheter that will be used later for the dilatation. Depending on which coronary artery is to be dilated, the cardiologist chooses either a "right" or a "left" pre-shaped guiding catheter. With the help of the x-ray camera, the cardiologist directs the guiding catheter toward the aortic root (the portion of the aorta near the heart) and into the opening of the coronary artery. (See figure 61).

When the guiding catheter is in the proper position, the cardiologist threads the thinner dilatation catheter through it. The dilatation catheter has a tiny (but very strong) balloon at its tip. With x-ray guidance, the dilatation catheter is slowly advanced into the coronary artery, until the balloon reaches the area of narrowing. The balloon is carefully positioned in the middle of the narrowing, and then inflated under pressure, thus compressing the soft plaque against the arterial walls (see figure 62). The inflation period usually lasts for about 30 seconds, and then the balloon is deflated.

The dilatation catheter is then pulled out, and a coronary angiogram is obtained by injecting dye through the guiding catheter. The cardiologist is thus able to visualize how much improvement has occurred following the dilatation. Sometimes, the balloon may have to be inflated and deflated several times, until the area of narrowing is satisfactorily dilated.

The angioplasty procedure generally lasts from 1 to 2 hours. As with cardiac catheterization, patients stay awake and fully conscious during the procedure and are generally able to watch the pictures on the television screen. The patient's cooperation is often needed during the procedure. The patient may be asked to take a deep breath and hold it for few seconds. Other times he may be asked to cough several times, in order to make his heart beat faster.

Coronary balloon angioplasty is not a painful procedure, although some discomfort may be reported during the manipulation of the catheters in the groin (or arm). The advancement of the catheters inside the blood vessels is painless. During the period of inflation of the balloon there is, as can be expected, a temporary obstruction of the coronary artery, leading to complete stoppage of blood flow to the heart muscle. This may result in symptoms of chest pain (angina). The discomfort, however, is only transient, and usually subsides shortly after deflation of the balloon.

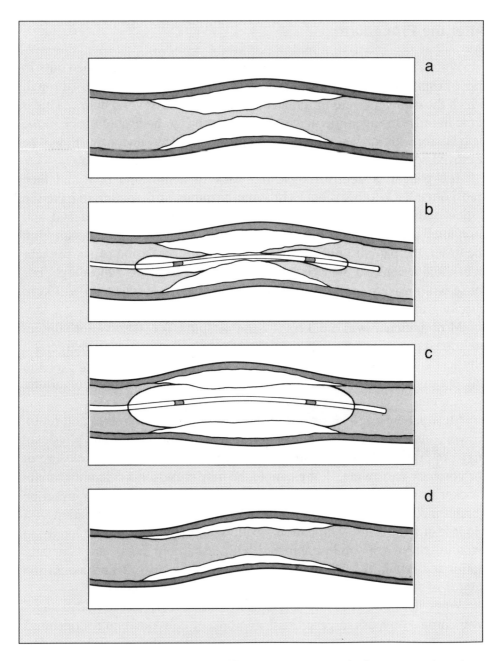

Figure 62. The basic steps of balloon angioplasty: a) A cross section of the narrowed coronary artery showing the plaque. b) The balloon is positioned in the middle of the narrowing. c) The balloon is inflated under pressure, compressing the plaque against the arterial wall. d) After the narrowing is satisfactorily dilated, the balloon is pulled out.

After the Procedure

When the angioplasty procedure is over, the catheters are pulled out. In most hospitals, it is now routine to leave the introducer sheath (through which the catheters were introduced) in the groin for several hours. This is done in order to save time in case the patient has to be brought back to the cath lab for additional emergency dilatations. The introducer sheath will be removed several hours later, when the patient is considered stable.

The patient is gently transferred back to a movable bed, and then transported back to his room. (In some hospitals, it is routine to have the patient moved to the intensive care unit, where he can be watched and monitored more closely). Following removal of the introducer sheath from the groin, the patient will remain lying in bed for a period of six to eight hours, and a sand bag will be applied to the area to prevent bleeding. The nurse will measure the blood pressure at frequent intervals, and will keep checking the groin, to insure that no bleeding has occurred.

Most patients will be kept in the hospital for observation for an additional period of one or two days. At some point before discharge, the physician will discuss with the patient and his family the results of the angioplasty procedure and will also give specific instructions regarding medications to be taken, physical activity, and diet.

Most patients will be able to resume their normal activities and return to work just a few days after discharge from the hospital. The physician may prescribe certain medications that will lessen the risk of re-closure of the coronary narrowing. For example, he may prescribe a calcium channel blocker to prevent spasm of the coronary artery. He may also prescribe certain medications (such as aspirin) that help prevent the formation of a blood clot at the site of dilatation. Follow-up diagnostic tests, such as an exercise stress test (often combined with a thallium scan), are generally performed within a few days after the procedure, in order to assess the degree of functional improvement resulting from the dilatation.

When feasible, coronary angioplasty has several distinct advantages over coronary bypass surgery. First, angioplasty does not require "opening" of the chest, and does not necessitate general anesthesia. Secondly, the recovery period is much shorter, and patients are generally discharged only a day or two following the procedure. Finally, hospital and surgical costs are usually reduced, sometimes dramatically.

Possible Risks and Complications

As with any other invasive procedures, coronary balloon angioplasty is associated with a certain degree of risk. As we have seen, the angioplasty procedure involves several steps, including insertion of a catheter into the body (catheterization), injection of dye into the coronary arteries (angiogram), and dilatation of the coronary artery lesion. Each one of these steps may be associated with certain complications. The complications (both minor and major) associated with cardiac catheterization and coronary angiography are relatively infrequent (see Chapter 10).

Complications encountered during coronary angioplasty generally result from the dilatation of the narrowing itself. When the balloon is inflated inside the coronary artery, it compresses the fatty plaque against the walls of the artery, thus allowing a better blood flow. At the same time, however, the balloon overstretches the walls of the artery, invariably causing a certain degree of injury to the thin innermost layer of the artery.

This injury to the arterial wall generally heals, over a period of days or weeks. In some cases, however, the injury leads to sudden blockage of the coronary artery and obstruction of the blood flow. If the obstruction cannot be reversed and coronary blood flow restored promptly, it may eventually result in myocardial infarction, that is, irreversible damage to the heart muscle. Sometimes the only way to restore the blood flow and prevent a myocardial infarction is to have the patient undergo emergency coronary bypass surgery.

Even when performed by an experienced physician, the risk of developing a major complication (such as a myocardial infarction or the need to have an emergency bypass surgery) during an angioplasty procedure is approximately 5 percent. The risk of dying as a result of the procedure is around 0.5 percent. In other words, 5 out of 100 persons undergoing coronary angioplasty may suffer a major complication, and 5 out of 1000 may die from it. This risk may seem high but, once again, we must not forget that most patients who require these procedures have significant coronary artery disease and are therefore at risk of developing a myocardial infarction unless properly treated.

Because of these potential risks, coronary angioplasty should be reserved only for selected patients. Before recommending such a major procedure, the cardiologist must weigh the benefits to be gained from angioplasty against the possible risks to the patient. He must inform the patient about the potential benefits to be derived from the procedure, the other alternatives (such as medical therapy or coronary bypass surgery, if appropriate), and the possible risks involved.

Results of Coronary Angioplasty

The primary goal of coronary balloon angioplasty is to dilate the area of narrowing and improve the coronary blood flow to the heart muscle. A coronary angioplasty is considered "successful" when there has been a satisfactory reduction in the degree of narrowing, as documented by a coronary angiogram (performed soon after the dilatation). When patients are carefully selected and the angioplasty is performed by a skilled physician, the success rate is around 80 percent.

Failure of coronary angioplasty, that is, the inability to dilate the artery, may occur for various reasons. In some cases, for example, it is impossible to reach the area of narrowing with the balloon catheter, because of sharp bends in the coronary arteries. Other times, it is possible to reach the area of narrowing, but then it is impossible to cross the tight narrowing with the balloon. In some cases, finally, it is possible to cross the lesion with the balloon, but the lesion cannot be dilated despite multiple inflations. This is most frequently seen when the plaque is heavily calcified and hardened and thus cannot be compressed against the arterial walls.

Re-closure of the coronary narrowing occurs in about 30 percent of those cases that were initially successful. When re-closure does occur, it generally happens within 3 to 6 months after the angioplasty procedure. Patients may develop a recurrence or worsening of their angina symptoms. Because of the relatively high rate of re-closure, many cardiologists perform a routine exercise stress test (usually with a thallium scan) in the months following the procedure. The test may detect evidence of insufficient coronary blood flow (ischemia) even in patients without symptoms. In case of re-closure, a second angioplasty is often recommended. The success rate in patients undergoing a repeat angioplasty is generally higher than in patients undergoing their first angioplasty.

Indication for Coronary Angioplasty

As we have seen, coronary balloon angioplasty has several advantages over coronary bypass surgery. Unfortunately, however, it has several technical limitations. The angioplasty procedure, for example, can be extremely difficult in patients with tortuous (curved) coronary vessels, where the lesion is located after sharp bends. In patients with long-standing disease, the plaque may have calcified and hardened, rendering the dilatation of the lesion extremely difficult.

In some patients, the dilatation is technically feasible, but the potential risk to the patient may be too high. In patients with severe narrowing of the left main coronary artery (before it divides into the two left branches), for example, a large amount of heart muscle could be at jeopardy in case of a complication. In these patients, a sudden closure of the lesion during angioplasty may result in a massive myocardial infarction and probable death within minutes or hours. For this reason, most cardiologists will not recommend an angioplasty in patients with left main coronary artery disease, but will rather refer the patient for coronary bypass surgery, which is relatively safer in such a case.

Patient selection for coronary balloon angioplasty is based on the angiographic findings and the nature of the clinical manifestations:

• On the basis of the coronary angiogram, the "ideal" candidate for angioplasty is a patient with the following findings: a significant and distinct "lesion," that is noncalcified (and thus compressible), involving a single coronary artery, and located proximally (near the origin of the coronary artery).

• Based on the clinical manifestations, candidates for coronary angioplasty should have symptoms of angina, or at least evidence of inadequate blood flow to the heart muscle (ischemia) documented by an exercise stress test (with or without a thallium scan).

Since its introduction in the late 1970s, the technology of coronary angioplasty has been constantly refined, and the physicians' skill and experience have improved tremendously. As a result, today's patient selection criteria have expanded, allowing additional groups of patients to be treated by this procedure.

Some cardiologists, for example, now perform coronary angioplasty in patients with more than one lesion in a single vessel, or in patients with several distinct lesions in more than one vessel. Other times, coronary angioplasty may be performed in the setting of an acute myocardial infarction, soon after the clot has been dissolved with streptokinase (see Chapter 14). Finally, coronary angioplasty may sometimes be used to dilate a narrowing of bypass vein grafts in patients who previously underwent coronary bypass surgery but later developed new angina symptoms.

When successful, coronary angioplasty can bring dramatic reduction in the frequency and severity of angina symptoms. There is often significant amelioration and even normalization of the exercise stress test. Such an improvement has persisted in many patients through follow-up periods of several years. Despite these promising results, however, coronary angioplasty cannot (and will not) replace coronary bypass surgery, and should therefore be performed only in carefully selected patients. At the present time, about 30 percent of the patients who are candidates for bypass surgery can benefit from this less invasive procedure.

24 **Coronary Bypass Surgery**

The purpose of coronary bypass surgery is to restore the flow of blood to areas of the heart muscle that receive an inadequate amount of blood and oxygen as a result of narrowing of the coronary arteries. Since its introduction in the late 1960s, coronary bypass surgery has gained increasing popularity as an effective treatment for patients with coronary heart disease, and symptoms of angina.

The objective of bypass surgery is not to remove the blockage, but rather to create a detour ("bypass") that lets blood go around the blockage. The operation does not "cure" coronary artery disease, but it relieves angina symptoms by improving the blood supply to the heart muscle.

To accomplish a bypass, a segment of a vein from the patient's leg is removed to be used as a vein graft. The vein is then attached at one end to a small opening made in the aorta (the major artery from which the coronary arteries originate) and the other end is sewn to an opening created in the coronary artery, beyond the narrowing or blockage. With the vein graft in place, blood can flow freely from the aorta into the coronary artery, beyond the blockage. (See figure 63, page 313).

Before the Operation

Before a coronary bypass operation can be performed, the candidate must first undergo cardiac catheterization and coronary angiography. These invasive studies are crucial in answering several important questions, such as: What is the degree of narrowing of the coronary arteries? What is the exact location of the narrowings ("lesions")? How many coronary arteries are involved? Is the pumping function of the heart compromised?

Only after reviewing the findings of these studies is the cardiologist able to accurately diagnose the underlying condition and assess its severity. By combining these findings with the clinical facts obtained previously (history, physical examination, and noninvasive tests), he can get an overall picture of the patient's problem. Only then will he be able to make an informed decision regarding the best approach to the problem. Although it is usually the cardiologist who will recommend the surgery to the patient, the evaluation process often involves combined efforts of the primary doctor (internist), the cardiologist, and the cardiac surgeon.

After a decision on whether or not to recommend surgery has been made, it is generally the cardiologist's role to explain the nature of the problem to the patient and his family, and to suggest what he believes is the best approach to the problem. If he feels, for example, that bypass surgery is the best approach, he should also present the other available alternatives (such as medications or coronary balloon angioplasty) and describe the benefits as well as the risks of these methods of treatment.

In some cases, when there is a doubt as to whether an operation should be performed, an additional consultation ("second opinion") may be advisable. This need most commonly arises when the patient or family have concerns or doubts about whether the operation is really necessary. Other times, especially when the indication for surgery is "borderline," it may be the cardiologist himself who will suggest a second opinion; in fact, a competent physician is usually more than willing to share the responsibility of such an important decision with another colleague. Today, an increasing number of insurance companies encourage their clients to seek a second opinion prior to any elective surgery, and will fully cover the expense.

If, after discussing the matter with his physician, the patient feels comfortable with the recommendations, then a second opinion is probably not necessary. If, on the other hand, there is any doubt as to whether the operation is indicated, then an additional consultation is appropriate. It should be kept in mind that a second opinion is not necessarily better than a first opinion; actually, a conflicting opinion may only make matters more confusing! In any event, whether there is agreement or disagreement, the final decision ultimately rests with the patient.

After the patient has accepted the recommendations and has agreed to undergo surgery, it is time to select the cardiac surgeon. The success of cardiac surgery depends to a great extent upon the skill and competence of the surgeon and his surgical team. Consequently, choosing the right surgeon is an important decision. Most patients have a great deal of confidence in their cardiologist and will leave the choice of surgeon to him. Other patients, however, may prefer to participate in the selection of the doctor who will perform the operation. In either case, some of the basic questions that should be considered are: the qualifications and competence of the surgeon; his reputation among physicians and patients in the community; and the number of operations he regularly performs.

The initial meeting between the patient and the cardiac surgeon (the "consultation") takes place either at the surgeon's office or at the hospital. Prior to the consultation, the cardiac surgeon would have had the opportunity to discuss the case with the cardiologist and to review the findings of the various diagnostic studies. During the consultation, the surgeon will explain what the bypass surgery involves and will discuss the potential benefits and possible risks from the operation. This is a good time for the patient to raise questions and discuss any concerns he might have regarding the operation and its outcome.

Preparation for Surgery

Patients are usually admitted to the hospital a day or two before surgery, so that routine preoperative tests can be performed. After the admission formalities have been completed, the patient is escorted to his room in the cardiovascular unit. A nurse from the unit will welcome the patient, familiarize him with the hospital routine, and then take his vital signs (pulse, blood pressure, respiration, and temperature).

At some point before surgery, the patient is asked to sign a *consent form,* a legal document that gives permission for the surgeon to perform the operation. "Informed consent" means that the patient is fully aware of the potential benefits and possible risks of the surgery before he agrees to it. By signing the consent form, the patient essentially accepts legal responsibility for the outcome, to the extent that he has been so informed.

Over the next day or two, patients go through a series of *routine preoperative tests.* Blood samples are drawn and processed in the hospital laboratory, to determine the blood count and to assess the function of the body's systems (such as the kidneys, liver, and endocrine glands). Another sample of blood is typed and cross-matched so that if blood is required for transfusion (during or after the operation), the type of blood transfused will be compatible with the patient's own blood type. A chest x-ray is taken in the x-ray department, and an ECG is performed in the patient's room.

Pulmonary functions studies, performed by a respiratory therapist, are generally part of the preoperative evaluation. During these studies, the patient is asked to blow forcefully into a small plastic tube attached to a machine that measures the capacity of the lungs and the force of the exhaled breath. Learning proper breathing exercises and coughing techniques is important for all patients undergoing cardiac surgery. Although breathing and coughing have been natural functions for a lifetime, these functions will not be as easy following the operation (after the lungs have been exposed, and the chest bone has been divided and later wired together). During the immediate postoperative period the patient will be asked to cough frequently in order to clear his lungs of secretions and to prevent the development of pneumonia. Clearly, it is easier to learn these techniques before the surgery than following it.

A very important part of the preparation for heart surgery is *emotional support.* A diagnosis of heart disease and impending heart surgery often have a significant emotional impact on the patient and his family. Although patients do react differently, the experience is almost always associated with a certain degree of apprehension, anxiety, and fear. Most hospitals have trained personnel on staff (nurses, psychologists, social workers) who are aware of the need to discuss feelings and concerns.

Another important aspect of the preparation for cardiac surgery is *patient education.* Many heart surgery teams have a patient educator (usually a specially trained nurse), whose role is to explain to the patient what can be expected before and after the operation. The educational process generally begins on the first day of hospitalization and continues after the surgery and throughout the early recovery period. Before the patient is discharged home, the nurse-educator will also provide specific instructions (regarding activity, diet, medications, etc.), in order to ease the transition between the hospital and home.

On the day prior to surgery, the patient is visited by the *anesthesiologist,* the doctor who will be responsible for the anesthesia (putting the patient to sleep) during the operation. The anesthesiologist will discuss his part in the surgery and will answer any questions the patient might have.

On the evening before surgery, the patient is *"prepped"* (cleansed and shaved) for the operation. He is asked to shower and wash his entire body with a sponge containing an antiseptic soap. Then, the patient's chest, groins, and legs will be shaved. Removing hair from the body not only is an important measure that ensures a sterile operative area during surgery, but also will make removal of the adhesive bandages much easier.

No later than 10 p.m., a light snack may be offered. From then on, the patient is kept strictly on "nothing by mouth." The only exception is the sip of water taken to swallow the sleeping medications that are given before bedtime, to ensure that the patient will sleep well despite his apprehension regarding the impending surgery.

The Bypass Operation

It is usually early in the morning when the slightly sedated patient is wheeled on a movable bed into the *operating room.* Just before being put to sleep, the patient is generally able to observe the surroundings.

Located in the center of the room is the operating table, mechanically adjustable to any height and angle, providing the surgeon with maximum access to the operative site. The overhead lights are of high intensity and can be positioned to give the best illumination of the operating field. At the foot of the operating table are the various instruments that will be needed during the surgery. Sophisticated electronic monitors will display the various physiological data (such as the ECG, blood pressure, and temperature) during the operation. Finally, in proximity to the operating table is the heart-lung machine (the "pump"), a large apparatus used to support the patient's life functions during certain stages of the operation.

The Surgical Team

As soon as the patient is wheeled into the operating room, he is transferred to the care of a group of highly trained professionals, known collectively as the surgical team. The success of heart surgery depends to a great extent upon perfect coordination and team work among the various members of the team.

The cardiac surgeon is the leader of the surgical team during the operation. As the operation proceeds, he will be performing and supervising the most critical aspects of the operation. The cardiac surgeon generally has two assistant surgeons whose role is to assist him during the operation. The anesthesiologist has the role of inducing general anesthesia (putting the patient to sleep) at the start of the operation, then maintaining the patient safely in state of deep sleep throughout the operation.

The scrub nurse has the task of setting up the sterile surgical instruments before the start of the operation. During the operation, she hands the surgeon the surgical instruments as they are needed. The circulating nurse is the operating room manager. With the exception of the operation itself, she has the responsibility for most of what takes place in the operating room. She oversees the proper function and safety of the operating environment. Finally, the pump technician (or perfusionist) is responsible for setting up the heart-lung machine before each operation, and for controlling the apparatus during the operation.

Before going into the operating room, all surgeons and nurses who will be directly involved in the operation must "scrub" for the surgery, in order to prevent contamination of the surgical "field" during the operation. The procedure includes a timed washing of hands and forearms with a disposable sterile brush soaked in special antiseptic solution. As soon as the surgeon enters the operating room, he is helped into a sterile gown and gloves by the scrub nurse.

During the Operation

A coronary bypass operation generally takes from 4 to 6 hours, depending on the patient's condition and the number of bypass grafts performed. The surgery itself can be separated into several stages: inducing general anesthesia; inserting the monitoring lines; removing the saphenous vein from the leg; opening the chest; connecting the heart-lung machine; operating on the heart; and closing the chest.

After being wheeled into the operating room, the patient is helped from the movable bed to the operating table. The anesthesiologist greets him, then inserts an intravenous line (a small needle to which a plastic tube is attached) into the patient's arm. It is through the intravenous line that anesthetic drugs are administered, in order to induce general anesthesia (putting the patient to sleep). From that moment on, the patient will be in a state of deep sleep and unaware of the activity around him.

When the anesthesiologist is certain the patient is deeply asleep, he can proceed with *insertion of the various monitoring lines and devices.* First, he inserts an endotracheal tube (breathing tube) through the patient's mouth into his trachea (windpipe), thus providing a direct channel to the lungs. The tube is attached to a respirator (breathing machine), which mechanically regulates breathing and assures an adequate supply of oxygen to the lungs throughout the operation.

Then, a urinary catheter (thin rubber tube) is placed in the bladder to drain and measure the urine output. This measurement provides an assessment of kidney function while the patient is asleep. Two additional "lines" are inserted, one into an artery in the wrist, and one into a large vein in the shoulder area. These lines are connected to electronic monitors that record the pressure in the arteries and veins and display the tracings continuously throughout the operation. Blood samples will be drawn from these lines periodically to ascertain that oxygen and other blood chemistry levels stay within the normal range. When the tubes and lines are all in place, the surgery can proceed.

To accomplish a bypass, a segment of saphenous vein from the patient's leg is removed, to be used later as a vein graft. Using a vein from the patient's own body eliminates the chance for rejection of the graft. The saphenous vein can be removed without risk since it is not essential for the circulation in the leg. The vein is extracted through a long incision that runs along the inside of the leg, from the lower calf to the thigh. After the vein has been removed, the incision is sutured and the leg is bandaged.

In some cases, the internal mammary artery, one of the arteries that carries blood to the inside of the chest wall, is used as a bypass vessel instead of (or in addition to) the saphenous vein.

While the assistant surgeon is busy removing the segment of saphenous vein from the patient's leg, another surgeon starts *opening the chest.* An incision is made down the center of the chest, and the sternum (breastbone) is divided vertically. The two halves of the sternum (connected to the rib cage) are gently separated and held open by a large metal retractor. This exposes the pericardium, that is, the thin sac that encloses and protects the heart. The surgeon then carefully cuts open the pericardial sac, exposing the beating heart.

In order for the surgeon to perform the delicate surgery on the heart itself, the heart action is stopped temporarily (for about an hour). During that period, when the heart is "quiet," the circulation is maintained with the *heart-lung machine.* This device is connected to the patient's circulation soon after the heart has been exposed. The oxygen-poor blood returning to the heart is diverted to the machine, where carbon dioxide is exchanged for oxygen. Then, the "fresh" oxygenated blood is returned by the machine into the patient's arterial system. Thus, the machine acts as a "heart" in that it pumps the patient's blood, and as a "lung" in that it exchanges carbon dioxide for oxygen. At the moment the machine completely takes over for the heart, the patient is said to be *"on the pump."*

To accomplish a *bypass graft,* a section of the aorta is isolated with a special clamp, and a small opening is made in the wall of the aorta. A segment of saphenous vein from the leg is then attached at one end to the small opening made in the aorta, and the other end is sewn to an opening created in the coronary artery, beyond the blockage (see figure 63). The procedure is repeated for each coronary artery to be bypassed. Patients may undergo "single," "double," "triple," or "quadruple" bypass surgery, depending on the number of coronary arteries or major branches that require a graft. When all grafts are in place, the clamp is removed from the aorta. Blood can then flow from the aorta, through the vein grafts, and into the coronary arteries beyond the narrowed or blocked area.

When the internal mammary artery is used instead of (or in addition to) the saphenous vein, the proximal (upper) end of the artery is kept untouched. The distal (lower) end of the artery is separated from the chest wall and then sewn to an opening created in the coronary artery. This way, blood flowing through the internal mammary artery is redirected into the coronary artery.

When all grafts are in place, the surgeon begins the process of taking the patient *"off the pump."* The heart may begin to beat spontaneously or may require a small electrical shock to get it started. During this procedure, the anesthesiologist, surgeons, and pump technician closely monitor the blood

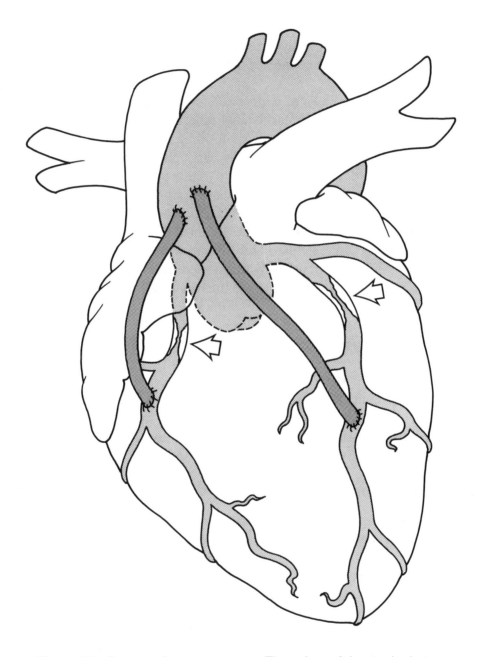

Figure 63. Coronary bypass surgery. The vein graft is attached at one end to a small opening made in the aorta, and the other end is sewn to an opening created in the coronary artery. Blood can now flow from the aorta into the coronary artery, beyond the blockage.

pressure and the ECG. With the heart beating on its own and the vital signs stable, the lines that have connected the patient to the heart-lung machine can be removed.

As the operation draws to a close, the surgeons begin the process of *closing the chest*. Two large plastic tubes (chest tubes) are inserted through the skin into the chest cavity in order to drain off any blood that might accumulate around the heart during the early postoperative period. The retractors that held the chest open are removed. Then, the sternum (breastbone) is brought back together with several small strands of stainless steel wire. These wires will remain in place permanently, ensuring that the bone will not shift when the patient moves about during the healing period. Finally, the skin is sutured closed and covered with a sterile dressing. The patient, still deeply asleep, is gently transferred from the operating table to a movable bed, then transported to the intensive care unit.

After the Operation

While still in a state of deep sleep, the patient is transferred to the Intensive Care Unit (ICU), where he will be closely monitored during the immediate postoperative period. Two or three days later, he will be transferred to the so-called step-down unit, where he will be able to increase his activities progressively.

The Intensive Care Unit

Following surgery, the patient is taken to a surgical intensive care unit that has been designed to provide close and continuous monitoring (surveillance) of all vital functions. The intensive care unit is staffed with specially trained nurses and other medical personnel familiar with the equipment and the various sophisticated devices in the unit.

Upon awakening from the anesthesia, generally within two or three hours after the operation, the patient may be disoriented, sore, and perhaps confused. He may hear a variety of sounds and voices, and see a blur of people in motion and a variety of machinery. It is generally the ICU nurse who will first talk to the patient, telling him that the surgery is over and that everything is fine. Over the next several hours, the patient may be visited by an array of people such as the anesthesiologist, the surgeon, the cardiologist, the ICU technicians, and close family members.

The ICU nurse is a highly trained nurse who is familiar with the equipment in the unit and who has the authority to take immediate action in emergency situations, even in the absence of a physician. During the patient's stay in the unit, the nurse will check his vital signs (such as blood pressure, pulse, breathing pattern, and temperature) at frequent intervals. Although this constant surveillance may become annoying for the patient, it is necessary for the proper assessment of his condition and the early detection of potential problems.

Above the patient's bed is the ECG monitor, an electronic device similar to a small television screen, that continuously assesses the patient's heart rate and rhythm during his entire stay in the ICU. Small adhesive electrodes are placed on the patient's chest and connected by wires to the ECG monitor and to a master monitor at the nurses' station. If an abnormal rhythm (arrhythmia) develops, the machine will sound an alarm that will alert the nurse. If the patient moves too suddenly or if a wire becomes loose, the alarm may go off accidentally.

Another vital piece of equipment, the respirator (breathing machine), stands close to the patient's bedside. The respirator is connected to the breathing tube, which was inserted in the patient's trachea at the beginning of the operation. The respirator brings oxygen to the lungs during the operation and during the immediate postoperative period, while the patient is not awake enough to breath on his own. During its function, the respirator makes a whooshing, bellowlike sound. If there is a problem in the circuit, the machine emits an alarm that will alert the nurse.

In order to prevent accumulation of secretions within the lungs, the nurse will suction the lungs through the breathing tube at frequent intervals. The process of suctioning is uncomfortable, but necessary to keep the lungs free from secretions that could lead to pneumonia. Because a portion of the breathing tube passes through the voice box, the patient cannot speak while the tube is in place. When the anesthesia has worn off and the patient is able to breathe on his own, the breathing tube is removed and the respirator turned off. This generally occurs within twelve hours after surgery.

The various lines and tubes that were inserted prior to the operation will remain attached to the patient during the immediate postoperative period.

The intravenous lines are used to administer fluids, glucose (sugar), blood, and various drugs. The arterial line (usually inserted in the wrist) is used to monitor the blood pressure, and to withdraw blood samples without any discomfort to the patient. The stomach tube, inserted through the nose, is used to suction the natural stomach secretions. The urinary catheter allows an accurate measurement of the urine output and helps in determining the functional status of the kidneys.

The chest tubes (usually two), which were inserted during the final stage of the operation, are used to drain any air or blood that tends to accumulate around the heart during the postoperative period. The chest tubes, coming through the chest wall, are attached to water-filled bottles that rest at the side of the bed. The closed drainage system emits a continuous gurgling sound. The chest tubes will be removed by the surgeon within two or three days after surgery, before the patient leaves the intensive care unit.

Prolonged immobility in patients recovering from any major surgery may lead to slowing of the circulation and formation of blood clots in the leg veins. Therefore, patients are encouraged to move as soon as feasible. The patient is asked to wiggle his toes, move the ankles, flex the feet, and bend the knees, all of which help the circulation in the legs. As soon as the breathing tube has been removed, the patient is helped to sit up in bed. Later, he will proceed to dangle his legs over the side of the bed for brief periods of time and then sit in a chair next to the bed.

In patients recovering from cardiac surgery, the respiration is rather shallow and the lungs tend to fill up with secretions that may lead to pneumonia. Patients are therefore encouraged to perform coughing exercises as soon as possible. The respiratory therapist may ask the patient to hug a pillow to support the incision during the cough and thus minimize the pain. He may also encourage coughing by gently clapping the patient's back. Patients are also encouraged to perform deep breathing exercises by blowing into special bottles or tubes several times a day. These exercises expand the sluggish lungs, clear the secretions, and prevent the development of pneumonia.

After surgery, some patients may complain of pain in the chest area, usually resulting from the surgical incision. Others are bothered by the incision in the leg through which the saphenous vein was removed. A sore throat may result from the endotracheal tube. Whatever its cause, pain can generally be relieved with a variety of pain medications that work quite effectively and are not addictive at the prescribed dosages.

Patients usually stay in the intensive care unit for a period of two to three days. During the first postoperative day, the breathing tube and the stomach tube are removed. The patient is then allowed to sit up in bed and a liquid diet is begun. By the second or third postoperative day, the arterial line comes out and the chest tubes are removed. Patients may then be bathed, sit in a chair, and even take a few steps around the bed.

The Step-down Unit

Once the tubes have come out and continuous monitoring is no longer necessary, the patient can be transferred to the step-down unit (also called intermediate care unit). The patient is allowed to walk around, first under supervision and then unassisted, and is encouraged to slowly increase his activities. Progressively, he becomes less dependent on others, and is able to attend to his personal needs.

Most step-down units have telemetry equipment. Patients wear a transistor-like device that continuously picks up the patient's ECG and relays the signals to a telemetry console nearby. Trained nurses sit at the central station to watch the tracings so that the patient's heart rate and rhythm are known at all times.

During the first few days after surgery, patients are encouraged to perform breathing and coughing exercises, first under supervision and then independently. As the lung function returns to normal, these exercises can be discontinued. Most centers also have physical therapy programs specifically tailored to the needs of postoperative heart patients. The physical therapist conducts daily exercises, such as walking around the unit, riding a stationary bicycle, and climbing stairs. Patients are provided with an exercise plan which can be followed at home after discharge.

Under normal circumstances, patients are discharged home about six to eight days after the operation. Prior to discharge, the patient and his family will be given instructions regarding the level of activity at home, the type of diet, and the various medications. In addition, the patient will be told what to expect during a normal recovery and what kind of potential problems could occur.

Postoperative Complications

Today, bypass surgery patients have far fewer postoperative complications than in the past. The technology of cardiac surgery has been constantly refined, and the skill and experience of the surgeons and nursing personnel have improved tremendously. In addition, several new sophisticated diagnostic techniques have made the preoperative evaluation of patients more accurate, thus improving the selection of patients who might benefit from surgery.

In spite of all reasonable precautions, however, problems and complications can still arise. Multiple factors play a role, but the most important one is the general health and lifestyle of the patient before the operation. Heavy smokers, for example, are more likely to develop lung complications, because their lungs have already been damaged from years of smoking. Markedly obese patients are at an increased risk of clot formation in the leg veins, because the circulation in their legs is more sluggish. Patients with severe coronary artery disease have a higher risk of myocardial infarction (heart attack), because a coronary blockage is more likely to occur during the operation. Finally, patients with a history of one or more previous myocardial infarctions are at a higher risk and generally take longer to recover, because their heart is already weaker going into surgery.

Patients recovering from cardiac surgery have a tendency to develop *lung complications.* During the immediate postoperative period, respiration is rather shallow and the lungs tend to fill up with secretions and mucus. If allowed to settle, these secretions can seriously interfere with the oxygen exchange. In addition, mucus plugs can block the bronchial tubes, leading to the collapse of small portions of the lungs, and eventually resulting in pneumonia. Therefore, even though it may be uncomfortable and painful, it is imperative for the patient to begin deep breathing and coughing exercises soon after the operation, in order to clear the lungs of secretions and prevent the development of pneumonia.

Another common problem in patients recovering from cardiac surgery are *vascular complications.* Following the operation patients have to lie immobile in bed for several hours, thus causing the circulation to become sluggish. The blood tends to pool in the leg veins, and small clots may begin to form, eventually resulting in inflammation and blockage of the leg veins (thrombophlebitis). The blood clots can become dislodged (they are then called emboli), travel through the bloodstream, and may end up in the lungs (pulmonary emboli), potentially causing serious breathing problems.

The best way to prevent vascular complications is by early mobilization during the immediate postoperative period. While lying in bed in the ICU, patients are encouraged to wiggle their toes, move the ankles, flex the feet, and bend the knees, all of which help the circulation in the legs. Soon after the breathing tube has been removed, patients are asked to sit in a chair at the bedside and even take a few steps. Another precautionary measure is the use of surgical stockings that put gentle pressure on the legs and keep blood from pooling in the veins, thus preventing clots from forming.

A small number of patients undergoing cardiac surgery may develop *neurological complications.* Most of these complications occur when arteries to the brain that were previously narrowed by plaques become blocked during the operation. Other times, the manipulation of the heart and aorta during surgery results in the formation of particulate matter (emboli) that can travel to the brain. The resulting blockage of small arteries in the brain deprives parts of the brain of oxygen and may result in transient or permanent damage (stroke). The manifestations of stroke are variable, and may include paralysis, speech difficulties, and confusion.

A myocardial infarction that occurs immediately before, during, or soon after the operation is termed a *perioperative myocardial infarction.* It is generally due to the sudden blockage of a previously narrowed coronary artery. It occurs in about 5 percent of patients undergoing bypass surgery. The perioperative infarction is usually so mild that it causes no symptoms. In most cases, it will not interfere with a normal recovery.

A common problem (not really a complication) following cardiac surgery is the occurrence of *incisional problems.* It takes several months for the breastbone to heal completely. During that period, patients may complain of aching, numbness, or itching in the area of the chest incision. Incisional pains can be relieved with a mild pain medication. Some patients develop inflammation of the incision sites in the chest or legs, marked by redness, swelling, and pain. These manifestations are generally short-lived, and improve within a few days. Less frequently, the incision gets infected, resulting in small amounts of pus draining from the site. The presence of incisional infection may require treatment with antibiotics.

Results of Bypass Surgery

The two main objectives of coronary bypass surgery are the relief of angina symptoms and the prolongation of life. Therefore, when evaluating the results of coronary bypass surgery, the two factors to be considered are: a) the effect of surgery on the relief of symptoms; and b) the effect of surgery on life expectancy.

The effects of coronary bypass surgery in achieving relief of symptoms are dramatic. Over 80 percent of patients suffering from angina who are operated upon will report substantial relief of their symptoms as well as a reduction in the use of antianginal drugs. Over half of these patients will become totally free of symptoms for prolonged periods of time. The results of exercise stress tests carried out before and after bypass surgery have substantiated the belief that true clinical benefit has been achieved, as opposed to only a subjective improvement.

The effects of bypass surgery on achieving the second objective, that is, the prolongation of life, are not as clear-cut. Whether or not surgery affects the long-term survival of patients with coronary heart disease is one of the most pressing questions in cardiology today, and can be answered only by comparing medically and surgically treated patients. This can be accomplished by the use of large-scale clinical trials, where patients are assigned at random to one of two groups, "medical" or "surgical," and patient survival in these suitably matched groups is compared.

Although some controversy still exists, there is general agreement among physicians that coronary bypass surgery improves longevity in several subsets of patients with coronary heart disease. Studies have shown, for example, that bypass surgery does prolong life expectancy in patients with significant narrowing of the left main coronary artery (before it divides into the two "left" coronary arteries). It has also been shown that surgery probably improves longevity in patients with significant coronary lesions in the proximal portion (that is, near the origin) of at least two of the three major coronary arteries.

Patients with a significant narrowing in a single coronary artery, on the other hand, generally have a good prognosis on medical treatment alone, and bypass surgery does not appear to improve their life expectancy (although it usually improves the symptoms).

On the average, elective (non-emergency) coronary bypass surgery is associated with an operative mortality of about 2 percent. In other words, out of every 100 patients undergoing surgery, two patients may die during the operation or during the early postoperative period. With emergency bypass surgery, the operative mortality can be as high as 10 percent. In general terms, the operative risk depends on the patient's general medical condition and on the presence of associated conditions (such as chronic lung disease or kidney disease). The operative mortality from bypass surgery differs among the various medical centers, suggesting that the experience and skill of the cardiac surgeon and his surgical team play a decisive role in determining the outcome.

Despite an initially successful operation, a number of patients will eventually develop recurrence of angina. Most frequently, the cause for chest pain is the progression of the preexisting coronary artery disease in the native (natural) arteries. As mentioned previously, the bypass grafts do not "cure" the disease, but merely create a detour that lets blood go around the blockage. In the meantime, the atherosclerotic plaques continue to build up as time goes on, especially if certain preventive measures (smoking cessation, diet, and exercise) are not taken.

Less frequently, recurrence of chest pain is due to the occlusion of the bypass graft(s). The closure of one of the grafts does not mean that the other grafts will also close. Actually, one graft may close and the others may remain open for life. Graft closure generally occurs when the recipient native coronary artery was too small (therefore making the grafting technically difficult), or when the disease simply progressed beyond the graft site. The development of atherosclerotic plaques in the vein graft occurs sometimes, but the process is generally very slow and may take years to build up to the point of significantly narrowing the graft.

General Indications for Bypass Surgery

Considerable controversy still exists regarding the specific indications for bypass surgery. Despite several large scale studies performed over the past decade, there is no specific formula upon which all physicians agree that will clearly determine who is a candidate for surgery and who is not.

The more "aggressive" physicians take the position that because coronary atherosclerosis is a progressive obstructive disease that will eventually result in myocardial infarction or sudden death, coronary bypass operation represents a logical solution. The more "conservative" physicians, on the other hand, hold that the complications, discomfort, and cost of the operation outweigh the questionable improvement in survival.

The truth probably lies somewhere between these two opposing views. There is now a general agreement that surgery is indicated to improve the "quality" of life in most patients who have disabling angina symptoms despite optimal medical therapy. There is disagreement, however, regarding the surgical indications for improving survival, that is, for increasing the "quantity" of life.

Two major factors are to be considered before a decision whether or not to recommend surgery can be made: a) the severity of symptoms and degree of disability; and b) the number, location, and severity of the coronary "lesions" as demonstrated by coronary angiography. Based on the above information, it is then possible to define several subgroups of patients that will most likely benefit from the bypass operation:

• Patients with persistent disabling symptoms of angina despite optimal doses of antianginal medications, and the presence of at least one critically narrowed coronary artery.

• The presence of significant narrowing of the left main coronary artery (before it divides into the two "left" coronary arteries), even if the symptoms can be controlled with medical therapy.

• The presence of significant coronary lesions in the proximal portion of at least two of the three major coronary arteries, when signs of ischemia (inadequate blood flow to the heart muscle) can be induced during an exercise stress test.

Obviously, these are only general broad guidelines. Patients with a condition as varied and complex as coronary heart disease cannot be treated according to a simple formula! There will always be patients at the "border" between those who do and those who do not possess the indications for coronary bypass surgery. Today, in addition, a certain number of these patients may benefit from a less invasive procedure, namely coronary balloon angioplasty (see Chapter 23).

Other variables that must be taken into consideration before recommending bypass surgery include the patient's general medical condition, his age, and his personal preference, as well as the experience and skill of the cardiac surgeon and his surgical team.

The decision process should involve combined efforts of the primary doctor (usually an internist), the cardiologist, and the cardiac surgeon. The eventual benefits from the surgery should be weighed against the possible risks, and the different options (such as medical therapy or coronary balloon angioplasty) should be clearly presented to the patient and his family.

Recovery: After Bypass Surgery

The recovery period allows patients to regain their strength and stamina. It also provides the most favorable condition for the healing process of the surgical incisions. Most patients are expected to recover and get back to normal within two to three months. However, the extent of the surgery, the rate of healing, and the general strength and stamina vary from patient to patient. Consequently, the time it takes to recover will also vary.

Except for the care of the surgical incisions, the guidelines for patients recovering from cardiac surgery are generally similar to the guidelines given to patients recovering from a heart attack. (For more information on recovery, see Chapter 25).

Care of the Surgical Incisions:

• By the time you leave the hospital, the chest incision should be fairly well healed. The chest bone may still be tender and the incisional area may at times become swollen. It usually takes six to eight weeks for the chest incision to heal completely.

• If healing is normal, you will probably get permission to take a shower or a bath at home. Wash your incision gently with mild soap and water and pat it dry with a towel.

Continued

• Pain in the area of the chest incision is fairly common during the early recovery period. Your physician will probably prescribe pain medications to relieve the discomfort. The pain will gradually decrease over a period of several weeks or months. In some patients, the pain may worsen during rainy days or damp weather.

• During the first few weeks after bypass surgery, it is not uncommon for the leg (from which the saphenous vein was removed) to become swollen. Your surgeon may recommend surgical stockings (tightly woven elastic knee-length hose) that will support the leg without interfering with the circulation. Their gentle compression will help to prevent fluid from accumulating.

• In addition, as often as possible you should elevate the leg from which the vein was removed. One way to do this is to place the leg on an opposing chair when sitting. Another method is to lie down with the leg supported on a pillow, for about an hour, several times a day. This will help to keep blood from pooling and the leg from swelling.

• Driving is usually not permitted for a period of about six weeks. If an accident (or sudden stop) occurs before the healing process is complete, the contact between the steering wheel and the chest can cause severe injury to the breastbone. At the beginning, drive the car for short periods of time (less than half an hour), preferably on city streets. Several weeks later, you will be allowed to drive for longer periods, and on the freeway. Do not forget to use seat belts!

• Call your physician if you develop problems in the area of the surgical incision, such as oozing, drainage, swelling, redness, or pain. A slight fever is not uncommon during the first week at home. If the fever is persistent or significant (over 100 degrees), or if you develop shaking chills, this may be a sign of infection. Call your physician and discuss the problem with him.

Part Five

LIVING WITH HEART DISEASE

25 Recovery and Lifestyle Adjustments

The rehabilitation of the patient with heart disease involves two basic stages: a) recovery from the acute cardiac event (such as a heart attack or cardiac surgery); and b) lifestyle adjustments, which include risk factor modification and psychological adjustment. Some cardiac patients may be referred to a formal cardiac rehabilitation program, which combines supervised exercise sessions, patient education, and counseling.

Recovery: After a Major Cardiac Event

After a heart attack, the body sets out to repair the injured heart muscle. Although the damaged area will never be a functioning muscle again, it will form into scar tissue which will maintain the integrity of the ventricular wall. The healing process, during which scar tissue replaces the injured heart muscle, requires about six to eight weeks.

The purpose of reduced physical activity during the recovery period is to provide the most favorable circumstances for the healing process. The purpose of a gradual progression of activity is to counteract the weakening effects of bed rest and inactivity.

Following the discharge from the hospital, it takes about two to three months for most patients to get back to "normal." However, the severity of the infarction, the rate of healing, and the general strength and stamina vary from patient to patient. Consequently, the time it takes to recover will also vary. A previously healthy individual who suffers a small infarction, for example, might be able to return to full activity within a month. A person with various health problems who suffers a large infarction, on the other hand, may require a recovery period of three to four months.

After coronary bypass surgery, the recovery period provides favorable conditions for the healing process of the surgical incisions. Most patients are expected to recover and get back to normal within a period of two to three months. However, the extent of surgery, the rate of healing, and the general strength and stamina vary from patient to patient. Consequently, the time it takes to recover will also vary.

Guidelines for Recovery

The following pages offer general guidelines for patients recovering from a heart attack or from coronary bypass surgery. Except for the care of the surgical incisions (see page 323), the guidelines for patients recovering from bypass surgery are essentially similar to those given to patients after a heart attack. Since the rate of recovery varies from patient to patient, these are only general guidelines. If any questions or concerns arise, it is best to contact the physician for more specific and detailed instructions.

Daily living activities:

• You can expect to feel tired during the first few weeks after the heart attack (or bypass surgery). This feeling of fatigue and lack of energy will eventually subside.

• The increase in your activities should be gradual. Be sure to slow down or stop the activity when you feel tired. Alternate your activities with periods of rest. And most importantly, use good judgment and "listen" to your body.

• You may climb stairs at home as part of your daily living activities. Take your time and rest if you become short of breath. Limit the number of trips up and down the stairs.

Continued

• Light walking, for short distances, is often recommended during the early recovery period. It improves muscle tone and promotes relaxation. It should be done in moderation and according to your physician's instructions. Avoid walking uphill, against a cold wind, or during hot and humid days. At the first sign of fatigue, stop and rest.

• During the first few weeks at home, light household activities (such as setting the table, preparing meals, washing dishes, dusting) are permissible, if you feel up to them.

• More strenuous activities, such as vacuuming, mowing the lawn, and bed-making should be avoided during that period. In general, it is best to avoid lifting anything heavier than ten pounds. This includes bags of groceries, which can be deceptively heavy.

• During the first two weeks at home, limit visits according to how you feel. Support from your family and friends can help you feel better, but you need rest and relaxation. Feel free to ask your visitors to leave, or excuse yourself when you begin to feel tired.

• Driving is generally permitted three or four weeks after a heart attack. Initially, drive the car for short periods of time (less than half an hour at a time), preferably on city streets. After several weeks, you will be allowed to drive for longer periods, and on the freeway.

• In patients recovering from bypass surgery, driving may not be permitted for a period of six weeks. If an accident (or sudden stop) occurs before the healing process is complete, contact between the steering wheel and the chest may cause severe injury to the breastbone. Do not forget to use seat belts!

• Get your physician's permission before making any travel plans. Travel should be leisurely and relaxed. Remember the restrictions about lifting heavy objects. Avoid carrying heavy luggages and suitcases. If necessary, get assistance or use a cart.

• If, while traveling, you have to sit for more than an hour at a time, the circulation in your legs may become sluggish. Walk the aircraft aisle or stop the car and walk a little, to keep the circulation moving.

Continued

Sexual Activity:

• Sexual intercourse is associated with a moderate increase in heart activity. As a rule of thumb, if you can comfortably climb two flights of stairs without difficulty, or walk three blocks briskly, you are probably ready to resume sexual intercourse.

• Resumption of sexual relations should, like all physical activities, begin gradually. In the early recovery period, sexual activity can be expressed with touching, holding, embracing and caressing. It is possible to experience closeness and love in any of these ways.

• When you feel ready for sexual intercourse, some positions will require a minimal amount of effort and therefore will be more comfortable for you. They include the "side-by-side" position and "active partner on top."

• Do not initiate sexual activity within two hours after a large meal or heavy drinking, because your heart works harder during the digestive process. It is best to pick a time when you are not tired or under emotional stress.

• Once begun, sex should be stopped if you begin to experience abnormal symptoms such as chest pain, shortness of breath, palpitations, or dizziness. Wait for these symptoms to subside before resuming activity. If symptoms are significant or persistent, notify your physician and discuss the matter with him.

Return to work:

• Most patients will be able to return to work after a heart attack (or bypass surgery). The timing usually depends on three considerations: the degree of damage to the heart, the rate of recovery, and the physical requirements of the job. People with sedentary or desk jobs often return to work in about two or three months. It usually takes longer for patients performing a more physical type of work.

• If feasible, try to resume your job functions slowly. For example, try to work for only a half day at first, and then gradually extend to a full

Continued

work day. If the job requires an excessive amount of physical labor, consider choosing a new occupation. If the job generates a great deal of mental tension and stress, you may want to reassess the situation before returning to work.

• If you cannot return to your former job because it is too strenuous, or because the employer has discharged you, consider vocational guidance for new work opportunities. You can contact the rehabilitation department of your state or local government.

Reducing Stress

• In patients recovering from a major cardiac event, emotional stress should be reduced, whenever possible. Excessive stress may cause acceleration of the heart rate, rise of the blood pressure, and overtaxing of the cardiovascular system.

• Be realistic and set practical goals. People who expect too much of themselves can get tense if things don't work out.

• Identify the activities you find satisfying in and of themselves, and focus on enjoying them, rather than on your performance or what rewards the activities might bring.

• Organize your time. Identify the time wasters. Leave yourself more time than you'll think you need to get somewhere or to accomplish something.

• Set priorities. Divide your tasks into three categories — essential, important, and trivial — and forget about the trivial.

• Get regular exercise. An exercise tune-up will increase your stamina, recharge your energy, and get rid of excess tension.

• Be sure to get enough sleep and rest because fatigue can reduce your ability to cope with stress. Eat regular, well-balanced meals with enough variety to assure good nutrition.

• Listen to your body — it will let you know when you are pushing too hard. When you get tired, slow down and take time to enjoy the world around you.

Continued

• Don't waste your anger on trivial matters, which you can do nothing about anyway, such as a delayed train, an inept waiter, or an abrupt salesperson.

• Learn good working habits. Clear your desk of all papers except those relating to the immediate problem at hand. Do things in the order of their importance.

• Learn relaxation techniques (such as muscle relaxation, deep breathing exercises, meditation, yoga, or biofeedback). Some of these techniques will require professional help to learn.

• On a tightly scheduled day, take a few minutes between appointments or activities for a relaxation break, such as stretching, breathing, or a short walk.

• Avoid the use of tranquilizers, sleeping pills, alcohol, or tobacco. These addictive substances may provide temporary relief from stress, but will not cure the underlying cause of the problem.

• Talk it out. Problems often seem much worse when you carry them all alone. Talking to a trusted friend or relative can help you sort things out and unload some of the burden.

• Finally, if stress and its effects do get out of hand, it's time to seek professional counseling or psychotherapy. Professionals in a position to help you include the family doctor, nurse, social worker, clergy, psychologist, and psychiatrist.

Cardiac Rehabilitation Program

A cardiac rehabilitation program is designed to provide optimal care for the cardiac patient throughout all phases of recovery. Candidates for the program are generally patients recovering from a major cardiac event, such as a heart attack or coronary bypass surgery. Occasionally, patients suffering from stable angina may also be referred to the program.

The goal of cardiac rehabilitation is twofold: a) restore the patient to optimal physiological, psychological, and vocational status, and b) prevent the underlying disease from progressing. This goal is achieved through supervised exercise sessions, patient education, and counseling. The program relies upon the expertise of a variety of skilled professionals, such as physicians, nurses, physical therapists, dietitians, and social workers.

The decision regarding participation in a cardiac rehabilitation program is made by the patient's personal physician. Upon referral to the program, the patient is evaluated by the program's physician and by the nurse coordinator, and then undergoes an exercise stress test. Based on the functional level attained during the stress test and the strength level observed during the first exercise session, each patient is given an individual prescription for training and conditioning.

The exercise sessions, taking place at the cardiac rehabilitation center, include a variety of exercises, such as treadmill walking, stationary bicycle, wall pulleys, dumbbells, and rowing machines. In some centers, Nautilus exercise equipment is available for strength training. The intensity, duration, and frequency of the exercise are increased during the course of the training program, as dictated by the patient's progress. During the supervised exercise session, ECG electrodes are attached to the patient's chest, so that the heart rate and rhythm can be constantly monitored. Patients are also taught to take their pulse while exercising, and are instructed not to let the heart rate exceed a specified upper limit.

The training sessions, each lasting for about an hour, are held three times a week for a period of three to four months. During that period, monthly progress reports are sent to the referring physician. At the end of this monitored phase of the program, the patient undergoes a repeat exercise stress test, to assess the progress made. Graduates of the program may join another fitness program (non-monitored), or may follow a program of regular exercise on their own.

Patient education is an important component of every cardiac rehabilitation program. Patients and their families are educated in the recognition, prevention, and treatment of heart disease. In addition, patients are enrolled in group discussions and lectures on a wide variety of topics that are of special interest to cardiac patients, especially topics on prevention of heart disease and risk factor modification.

The program may also offer counseling by trained personnel, during private or group sessions. The dietitian, for example, will provide specific instructions regarding proper diet and weight reduction. A psychologist (or social worker) will deal with the anxiety, depression, and denial that patients and their families often experience as a result of the illness.

Lifestyle Adjustments

Very often, people who have a heart attack or are diagnosed as having heart disease are both stunned and frightened. Although one out of five Americans at some point develops heart disease, most harbor the notion that "it won't happen to me." When it does happen, there is a tendency either to deny that anything is wrong or to move to the opposite extreme and become a "cardiac cripple." Other common reactions include apprehension, anxiety, anger, frustration, and depression. These feelings are common and are considered abnormal only if they are intense or last for too long.

Some patients accept their situation with determination and optimism. Others become very depressed or adopt a defeatist attitude. The two most important psychological factors in making a good recovery are: acceptance of the fact that one has a chronic disease, and a positive mental attitude. Professional counseling or group therapy may be appropriate and should be extended to spouses and other family members as well.

Although some adjustments may be required, most people with heart disease are able to lead a productive and relatively normal life. Even after a major heart attack, most survivors are able to return to work (depending on the nature of their job) and engage in pleasurable pursuits such as exercise and sex.

The presence of certain risk factors (such as smoking, high blood pressure, elevated blood cholesterol, and obesity) often lead to the continuing build-up of fatty plaques in the coronary arteries. It is therefore important that patients recovering from a heart attack (or bypass surgery) make some adjustments in their life style. The period of recovery is usually the best time to start making those changes, because it is when patient's motivation is the greatest.

Giving up smoking is mandatory for patients who smoke and have heart disease. Cigarette smoking is associated with an increased risk of developing coronary heart disease, chronic lung disease, and lung cancer. Smoking also leads to progressive decline of the respiratory function and reduction of exercise tolerance. In patients with angina, smoking causes acceleration of the heart rate and decline in the amount of oxygen in the blood, and may therefore result in increased frequency and severity of angina attacks. The recovery period following a heart attack or bypass surgery is surely a good time to stop smoking. However, the best time to give up the habit is now, before any real damage is done!

Alteration of eating habits should be part of the lifestyle adjustments. In patients with coronary heart disease, for example, a diet low in fat and cholesterol will slow down or may even prevent the build-up of fatty plaques within the walls of the coronary arteries. Achieving and maintaining a desirable body weight, by adjusting the caloric intake, is another important adjustment. In patients with symptoms of angina or heart failure, weight loss will result in reduction of the workload on the heart, and may therefore improve the symptoms.

All too often, heart attack patients assume that they can no longer engage in pleasurable activities, including athletics. This is not true, however, for the large majority of patients. In fact, regular exercise is now advised for most patients recovering from a major cardiac event. Besides improving cardiovascular fitness, regular exercise tends to lower the blood pressure; helps lose extra pounds; improves muscle tone and flexibility; helps in coping with stress, anxiety, and depression; and enhances a person's sense of well-being. Patients with heart disease should always consult their physician prior to starting an exercise program. When exercising, it is also important to use moderation and common sense, in order to avoid exercise-related risks or injuries.

For some patients, adjustments in daily living activities will be necessary. Strenuous activities should be modified if they constantly and repeatedly produce symptoms. Patients with angina, for example, should avoid activities that consistently induce chest discomfort. Many activities, such as shopping or climbing stairs need not be discontinued; often it is merely necessary to perform them more slowly, or to pause for brief periods of rest. In patients with symptoms of congestive heart failure, the degree of activity should be adjusted to the severity of the symptoms. Activities that produce shortness of breath and fatigue should probably be discontinued. If it is essential for these activities to be continued, they should be carried out more slowly, and should be interrupted with rest periods.

Most patients will be able to return to work after a major cardiac event. The normal stress of work is seldom dangerous to the heart. For some people, quitting work and staying home can be even more stressful, perhaps because of boredom, loneliness or a sense of uselessness. If the previous job requires an excessive amount of physical labor, or if it generates a great deal of mental tension and stress, it may be necessary to choose a new occupation. When choosing a new occupation, the amount of satisfaction one gets from the work should be one of the most important factors.

The majority of patients recovering from a heart attack or bypass surgery will be able to resume satisfying sexual activity. Though many people who have had a heart attack fear that sexual intercourse may be life-threatening, studies have shown that this is rarely true. Some positions require a lesser amount of effort and therefore may be more comfortable to the cardiac patient.

In patients with heart disease, especially in those recovering from a major cardiac event, emotional stress should be reduced, whenever possible. Excessive stress may cause acceleration of the heart rate, rise of the blood pressure, and overtaxing of the cardiovascular system. In patients with coronary heart disease, for example, emotional stress can bring on a variety of potentially serious conditions, such as angina, cardiac arrhythmias, and congestive heart failure. In patients with severe coronary disease, a heart attack can be sometimes precipitated as a result of upsetting life events, such as the loss of a loved one, a major threat to professional or financial status, or following an outburst of anger or joy.

Obviously, it may be impossible to eliminate stress completely from one's life. Also, a certain amount of stress often adds variety and spice to life. Stress management techniques (such as relaxation, regular exercise, biofeedback) may help reduce the impact of stressful events. Patients who are unable to cope with stress, and those who manifest excessive symptoms of anxiety, depression, or anger, can benefit from professional counseling, psychotherapy, or group therapy.

The existence of heart disease often puts significant strain on the patient's family life. After a major cardiac event, family members may be concerned about the immediate outcome. During the recovery period, the patient and his family may begin to worry about various things, such as medical bills, job status, and physical limitations. The spouse may have to take on new responsibilities that were previously shared. Often a patient's attitude toward his recuperation is reflected in the way his family and friends treat him. The spouse, for example, may overprotect the patient, generally out of fear and lack of understanding of the patient's condition.

This may reinforce the patient's feelings of anxiety, weakness, and incompetence. Therefore, the patient should not be left out of discussions and decision-making within the family circle. The real issues of family life are unavoidable, and the patient needs to take part in resolving them.

A major factor in living well with heart disease is a good doctor-patient relationship, based on effective communication and trust. The doctor must explain the nature of the heart condition in a language that the patient can understand, avoiding complex medical jargon. He should emphasize prevention and provide recommendations for risk factor modification. The doctor should alert the patient to symptoms that may indicate the need for a return visit. When prescribing a new medication, he should mention the possible side effects and provide for follow-up if necessary.

In order to claim a share in the decision-making, patients should educate themselves by reading educational materials and by asking appropriate questions. Patients must follow their doctor's instructions, take medications as directed, and report any symptoms and side effects. Finally, they must take the important preventive measures that only they can take, such as giving up smoking, eating a proper diet, and exercising regularly. People generally feel healthier when they understand what's happening to them, and when they realize they can promote their own health by making real changes in their lifestyles.

Patient Resources

American Heart Association

The American Heart Association is a voluntary, nonprofit health organization funded by private contributions. Its stated goal is to reduce early death and disability from heart disease, stroke, and related disorders. To achieve this goal, the AHA funds medical research, professional and public education, and community service programs.

Information regarding the type of services in specific localities may be obtained by contacting the local AHA chapters, or by writing to the national headquarters in Dallas:

American Heart Association
7320 Greenville Avenue
Dallas, Texas 75231

Mended Hearts

The Mended Hearts is a voluntary, nonprofit organization consisting of people who have had heart surgery, their family members, and other interested individuals. Specially trained members of the Mended Hearts visit patients in the hospital before or soon after heart surgery, in an effort to offer encouragement and assistance.

Information regarding specific activities can be obtained by calling the local Mended Hearts chapter, or by writing to:

The Mended Hearts, Inc.
7320 Greenville Avenue
Dallas, Texas 75231

Glossary of Medical Terms

The following glossary contains a selection of words and terms commonly used in the field of cardiology and medicine. Terms not listed in the glossary will often be found in the index.

Acute   Having a rapid onset, a short course, and pronounced symptoms.

Adrenalin (also called epinephrine)   One of the hormones produced by the adrenal glands. It constricts the small blood vessels, increases the heart rate, and raises the blood pressure.

Aneurysm   A ballooning-out of the wall of a heart chamber or a blood vessel, due to a weakening of the wall by disease or injury.

Angina (also termed angina pectoris)   Chest pain or discomfort due to inadequate supply of blood and oxygen to the heart muscle, resulting from the narrowing of one or more coronary arteries.

Angiography   A diagnostic technique that involves the injection of x-ray dye (contrast) into the heart chambers or blood vessels, thus providing a detailed picture of the inside of these structures. The record of pictures is called an angiogram.

Angioplasty   A technique used to dilate arteries at the point where they have become narrowed by a plaque.

Antianginals   Drugs used to relieve angina symptoms.

Antiarrhythmics   Drugs that help control or prevent cardiac arrhythmias.

Anticoagulants (commonly called "blood thinners")   Agents that retard the blood clotting process.

Antihypertensives Drugs that lower blood pressure.

Aorta The body's largest artery, it carries blood from the main pumping chamber (left ventricle) and distributes it to all parts of the body.

Aortic valve The valve through which oxygenated blood passes from the main pumping chamber (left ventricle) to the body's largest artery (aorta).

Arrhythmia Any deviation from the normal rhythm of the heartbeat.

Arterioles The smallest arteries, that result from repeated branching of the arteries. They conduct blood from the arteries to the capillaries.

Arteriosclerosis (commonly called "hardening of the arteries") A general term referring to the hardening and loss of elasticity of the arterial walls associated with the aging process. *See also* Atherosclerosis.

Artery A blood vessel that transports blood away from the heart to the rest of the body. An artery usually carries oxygenated blood, except for the pulmonary artery which carries unoxygenated blood to the lungs.

Atherosclerosis A form of arteriosclerosis in which, in addition to the hardening and loss of elasticity of the arteries, a fatty substance (plaque) forms on the inner walls of the arteries, causing obstruction to the flow of blood. *See also* Arteriosclerosis.

Atrium One of the two upper chambers of the heart. The right atrium receives unoxygenated blood from the body. The left atrium receives oxygenated blood from the lungs.

Auscultation The act of listening to sounds within the body, usually with a stethoscope.

Beta blockers Drugs that block the action of the beta receptors, the nerve endings that affect the heart rate and the force of contraction. They are used for the treatment and control of angina, high blood pressure, and certain cardiac arrhythmias.

Blood pressure The force exerted by the blood against the arterial walls, created by the heart as it pumps blood to all parts of the body.

Blood vessel A vein or artery.

Bradycardia An abnormally slow heart rate. Generally, anything below 60 beats per minute is considered bradycardia.

Calcium channel blockers   Drugs that block the calcium transport mechanism in blood vessels and heart muscle cells. They relax the walls of the coronary arteries, and thus prevent coronary spasm. They are used mainly for the treatment and prevention of angina.

Capillaries   Tiny, thin-walled blood vessels, forming a network between the arterioles and the veins. They facilitate the exchange of substances between the surrounding tissues and the blood.

Cardiac   Pertaining to the heart.

Cardiac output   The amount of blood pumped by the heart each minute.

Cardiologist   A specialist in the diagnosis and treatment of heart disease.

Cardiology   The study of the heart and its functions in health and disease.

Cardiomyopathy   A general term for diseases that involve primarily the heart muscle (myocardium).

Cardiopulmonary   Pertaining to the heart and lungs.

Cardiovascular   Pertaining to the heart and blood vessels.

Cardioversion   The application of very brief discharges of electricity across the chest wall and into the heart, in order to stop certain cardiac arrhythmias and allow the normal cardiac rhythm to take over.

Catheter   In cardiology, a thin and flexible tube that can be inserted into a vein or artery (in the groin or arm) then directed toward the heart. The progression of the catheter inside the body can be followed with the aid of x-ray equipment.

Catheterization   In cardiology, the process of introducing a thin and flexible tube (catheter) into a vein or artery then directing it toward the heart, for the purpose of examining the heart function.

Cholesterol   A fat-like substance that is found in meat, dairy products, and eggs. It is normally present in the blood. Too high a level of cholesterol is associated with an increased risk of coronary heart disease.

Chronic   Of long duration, or frequent recurrence.

Circulatory   Pertaining to the heart, blood vessels, and the circulation.

Coagulation   The process of changing from a liquid to a thickened or solid state. The formation of a clot.

Collateral circulation Circulation of the blood through nearby smaller vessels when a main vessel has been blocked.

Congenital That is present at birth.

Congestive heart failure A condition in which the weakened heart is unable to pump enough blood to maintain normal circulation. It leads to congestion of the lungs and retention of water.

Coronary Related to the coronary arteries, the blood vessels that supply the heart muscle with blood and oxygen.

Cyanosis A bluish discoloration of the skin, fingernails, and lips, due to insufficient amount of oxygen in the blood. It is seen in patients with certain types of congenital heart defects.

Defibrillation Termination of fibrillation. Usually refers to the treatment of ventricular fibrillation (a life-threatening arrhythmia) by the application of an electric shock (cardioversion).

Diastole In each heartbeat, the period during which the pumping chambers (ventricles) relax and fill with blood. The diastolic reading obtained in blood pressure measurement is the lower number.

Digitalis A drug that strengthens the force of contraction of the heart and slows down the rate at which it beats. Digitalis drugs are used in the treatment of congestive heart failure and in the management of certain cardiac arrhythmias.

Dilatation An enlargement of the heart chambers or blood vessels.

Diuretics Drugs that increase the flow of urine and excretion of body fluid.

Dyspnea Difficulty in breathing.

Echocardiography A diagnostic technique that utilizes ultrasound waves to visualize and examine the heart structures. The record of pictures is called an echocardiogram.

Edema Swelling of body tissue caused by a buildup of fluid.

Effusion Accumulation of fluid between body tissues or in body cavities.

Electrocardiography A diagnostic technique in which small metal discs (electrodes) are placed on the patient's chest, arms, and legs, for the purpose of recording the electrical activity of the heart. The resulting tracing is called an electrocardiogram (ECG or EKG).

Embolism The blocking of a blood vessels by a clot (embolus) carried in the bloodstream.

Embolus A bit of matter (generally a blood clot) which drifts unattached in the bloodstream until it lodges in a blood vessel and obstructs it.

Endocarditis Infection of the inner lining of the heart chambers (endocardium) by micro-organisms which have entered the bloodstream. In most cases, the infection involves the heart valves, leaving the rest of the endocardium unaffected.

Fibrillation Uncoordinated contraction or twitching of the heart muscle, resulting in an irregular heartbeat. It may involve the upper chambers (atrial fibrillation) or the lower chambers (ventricular fibrillation).

Heart attack *See* Myocardial Infarction.

Heart block An arrhythmia caused by disruption (either partial or total) of the cardiac electrical conduction pathway. This can lead to dissociation of the rhythms of the upper and lower heart chambers.

Heart failure *See* Congestive Heart Failure.

Heart murmur An abnormal whooshing sound that can be heard with a stethoscope, resulting from turbulence in the bloodstream. It generally represents a defective (narrowed or leaky) heart valve.

Heart-lung machine A machine through which the bloodstream is diverted for pumping and oxygenation during heart surgery.

Hemorrhage Abnormal bleeding and loss of blood.

High blood pressure *See* Hypertension.

Hormone Secretion from a gland transported by the bloodstream to various organs in order to regulate vital functions and processes.

Hyper- Excessive, increased.

Hypercholesterolemia An excess of cholesterol in the blood.

Hypertension High blood pressure. A condition characterized by an excessive amount of pressure within the arteries.

Hypertrophy Increased size and thickening of a muscle, thereby adding to the number of muscle units able to contract, and strengthening the force of contraction. It generally occurs in response to an increased workload.

Hypo- Insufficient, decreased.

Hypotension Low blood pressure.

Infarction An irreversible damage to an area of tissue as a result of a total blockage of the blood supply. *See also* Myocardial Infarction.

Insufficiency *See* Regurgitation

Ischemia A local, usually temporary, deficiency in oxygen supply to some part of the body, due to obstruction or constriction of the blood vessel supplying that part.

Kidneys The two organs that regulate salt and water metabolism, and remove waste products from the bloodstream. They filter the blood and eliminate wastes through production and secretion of urine.

Lesion In cardiology, the narrowing of a coronary artery seen on the coronary angiogram.

Lipid Fat or fat-like substance, such as cholesterol and triglycerides.

Lipoprotein A complex consisting of lipid (fat) and protein molecules bound together. Since lipids do not dissolve in the blood, they must circulate in the form of lipoproteins.

Lungs Two organs of spongelike tissue that participate in the respiration. They are vital to oxygenation of blood and expulsion of gaseous waste (carbon dioxide) from the body.

Mitral valve A heart valve through which blood passes from the left upper chamber (left atrium) to the main pumping chamber (left ventricle).

Murmur *See* Heart Murmur.

Myocardial infarction An irreversible damage to an area of the heart muscle, caused by a total blockage of a coronary artery.

Myocardium Heart muscle.

Nitrates Drugs that relax the walls of blood vessels, both veins and arteries, causing them to dilate. Used mainly in the management of angina.

Nitroglycerin A drug (a nitrate) that relaxes the walls of blood vessels, causing them to dilate. Used primarily for the treatment of angina attacks.

Obesity Excessive weight. Generally defined as a 20 percent excess over "ideal" body weight (based on one's age, height, and bone structure).

Occlusion In cardiology, the total closure of a blood vessel.

Open Heart Surgery Surgery performed on the heart while the patient's blood is diverted through a heart-lung machine — whether or not the heart itself is opened.

Orthopnea A condition in which there is difficulty in breathing except when sitting or standing upright.

Oxygen A gas that is essential for life. It is vital to energy-producing chemical reactions in the living cells of the body. Breathed into the lungs, it enters the bloodstream and is carried by the blood to the body tissues.

Pacemaker (also called sinus node) A small bundle of cells which generate tiny electrical impulses, setting the pace for the heartbeat. Artificial pacemakers are electronic devices that can substitute for a defective natural pacemaker by delivering electrical stimuli to the heart.

Palpitations An unpleasant awareness of the heartbeat. Often described as skipped beats or as a fluttering sensation.

Pericarditis Inflammation of the pericardium.

Pericardium A thin membrane sac that surrounds the heart.

Physiology The science that studies the functions of body organs.

Plaque In cardiology, the abnormal buildup of fatty deposits on the inner layer of an artery. Plaques reduce the internal diameter of the artery, and may lead to total blockage.

Platelets Tiny bodies in the blood that have an important function in the blood-clotting mechanism.

Polyunsaturated fats Fats so constituted chemically that they are capable of absorbing additional atoms of hydrogen. They are predominantly vegetable in origin, and are usually liquid at room temperature.

Potassium A essential mineral in the body that is necessary for muscles to contract. It often gets "washed out" in the urine by diuretic drugs.

Prognosis   Prediction or forecast of the probable course of a disease.

Prophylaxis   Prevention of disease. In cardiology, the use of antibiotics to prevent an infection of the heart valves.

Pulmonary   Pertaining to the lungs.

Pulmonary artery   The large artery that transports unoxygenated blood from the right pumping chamber to the lungs. This is the only artery in the body that carries unoxygenated blood.

Pulmonary circulation   The circulation that carries unoxygenated blood from the heart to the lungs. It includes the right heart chambers, the main pulmonary artery, and the smaller pulmonary arteries.

Pulmonary edema   A severe form of congestive heart failure. There is flooding of the air sacs in the lungs, producing severe shortness of breath.

Pulmonary embolism   A condition in which a blood clot (embolus), usually one formed in a vein of the leg, breaks loose and becomes lodged in one of the arteries in the lungs.

Pulmonic valve   A heart valve through which unoxygenated blood passes from the right pumping chamber (right ventricle) to the pulmonary artery, and to the lungs.

Pulse   The expansion and contraction of an artery which may be felt with the fingers. Most commonly felt at the wrist.

Rales   Moist crackling sounds that can be heard over the lower portion of the lungs, most commonly in patients with congestive heart failure.

Regurgitation (or insufficiency)   The backward flow of blood (leakage) through a defective valve.

Renal   Pertaining to the kidneys.

Respiration   Breathing.

Resuscitation   Restoration of breathing or heartbeat to one who is apparently dead or threatened with death.

Risk factors   Conditions and habits associated with an increased risk or likelihood of an individual developing coronary heart disease.

Rupture   A tearing or bursting of a part.

Saturated fats Fats so constituted chemically that they are not capable of absorbing additional atoms of hydrogen. They are predominantly of animal origin (meat, milk), and are usually solid at room temperature.

Septum A dividing wall between two chambers. The ventricular septum is located between the two ventricles; the atrial septum is located between the two atria.

Shock A condition resulting from inadequate circulation. It may be due to loss of blood or to extreme weakness of the heart pump. Shock is marked by low blood pressure, rapid pulse, paleness, and cold, clammy skin.

Shunt Diversion of blood between the two sides of the heart, due to the presence of an abnormal opening (hole) within the heart or near the heart.

Sinus node The natural pacemaker. A small bundle of specialized cells that generate tiny electrical impulses which spread from the upper to the lower heart chambers, setting the pace for the heartbeat.

Sinus rhythm The normal heart rhythm as initiated by the electrical impulses in the sinus node (the natural pacemaker).

Sodium An essential mineral that is necessary to keep fluids distributed in the body. Table salt (sodium chloride) is nearly half sodium.

Spasm A temporary contraction of a segment of the arterial wall.

Sphygmomanometer An instrument used to measure blood pressure.

Stenosis A narrowing or stricture of an opening or a valve.

Stethoscope An instrument that amplifies bodily sounds, used for listening to sounds within the body.

Stroke An interruption of the blood flow to the brain, causing damage to the brain. Depending on the severity and location of the stroke, it may result in partial or total paralysis, loss of speech, or death.

Syncope A fainting spell. A sudden loss of consciousness due to a temporary reduction of blood flow and oxygen supply to the brain.

Systemic circulation The general circulation, as opposed to the pulmonary circulation. It carries oxygenated blood to the entire body, except the lungs. It includes the left heart chambers, the aorta, and the peripheral arteries.

Systole   In each heartbeat, the period during which the pumping chambers (ventricles) contract and eject their blood content.   The systolic reading obtained in blood pressure measurement is the higher number.

Tachycardia   An abnormally fast heart rate.   Generally, anything over 100 beats per minute is considered a tachycardia.

Thrombosis   The formation of a blood clot (thrombus) that partially or completely blocks a blood vessel.

Tricuspid valve   The heart valve through which blood passes from the right upper chamber (right atrium) to the right pumping chamber (right ventricle).

Triglycerides   The most common type of lipid (fat) found in fatty tissue. As opposed to cholesterol, no definite correlation has been found between the blood level of triglycerides and the incidence of coronary heart disease.

Valve   A flexible structure that regulates the flow of blood within the heart. It allows the blood to circulate in only one direction, and prevents it from backing up.

Vascular   Pertaining to blood vessels.

Vasodilators   Drugs that lower the blood pressure by relaxing the wall of peripheral arteries, causing them to dilate.   They are used mainly for the treatment of high blood pressure.

Vein   Any one of the blood vessels that carry unoxygenated blood from all parts of the body back to the heart.

Ventricle   One of the two pumping (or lower) chambers of the heart.   The left ventricle (main pumping chamber) pumps oxygenated blood through the arteries to all parts of the body, except the lungs.   The right ventricle pumps unoxygenated blood through the pulmonary artery to the lungs.

Index